Surviv... g

Safe and effective prescribing is one of the pillars of medical practice but is much more complicated than it seems. Many new prescribers find prescribing extremely challenging, and a plethora of independent, multidisciplinary prescribers are also seeking guidance. However, pharmacology textbooks are rarely practical. They warn to 'take care when prescribing erythromycin to a patient on warfarin, as the INR may rise'. But what should the prescriber actually do?

Surviving Prescribing fulfils an important need by offering practical advice for real-world prescribing problems. The book complements existing educational resources but adds a new perspective. Written by experienced contributors from a variety of professional backgrounds, the content speaks directly to the problems routinely seen in hospital prescribing. And all in one pocket-sized volume.

Whether revising for the national Prescribing Safety Assessment, preparing for starting on the wards, or looking for a quick reference guide, this book is an essential companion.

Mayur Murali is an anaesthetic trainee and an alumnus of the National Medical Director's Clinical Fellowship at NHS England, London, UK. He has completed a Masters in Medical Education and is a Fellow of the Higher Education Academy.

Robert Shulman is an experienced clinical pharmacist specialising in critical care at University College London Hospitals NHS Foundation Trust, London, UK. He is joint author of *Handbook of Drugs in Intensive Care* (Cambridge University Press, 2019).

Hugh Montgomery is Professor of Intensive Care Medicine at University College London, UK, and a practising clinician. He is on the Council of the UK Intensive Care Society and has published over 500 scientific papers.

Wow. This is a phenomenal piece of work. Excellent for medical students, specialty trainees and anyone prescribing outside specialty. It acknowledges both the complexity and risks of prescribing and provides a framework that spans pre-clinical pharmacology and prescribing at the bedside. I wish this book had been written 20 years ago. It's chatty and readable and will be an invaluable resource to students and doctors alike.

Dr Chris van Tulleken, Honorary Associate Professor, UCL, London, UK

A valuable source of information and reference and a 'must read' text to support education and learning for prescribers in all health sectors.

Ian Bates, Professor of Pharmacy Education, UCL School of Pharmacy, London, UK

Surviving prescribing is a must have for new prescribers. An easy-to-use, practical guide to prescribing, it is full of useful tips and easy-to-remember acronyms, in a concise readable format. It will help the reader develop their knowledge of key therapeutic topics, calculation methods, serious drug interactions and electronic prescribing. The comprehensive content is primarily written for hospital-based prescribers though practitioners in care homes, general practice, domiciliary and other primary care settings will find much of the content useful too.

Nina L. Barnett, Consultant Pharmacist, London North West University Healthcare NHS Trust & NHS Specialist Pharmacy Service, and Visiting Professor, Kingston University, London, UK

Surviving Prescribing

A Practical Guide

Second Edition

Edited by

Mayur Murali
Anaesthesia Trainee, Imperial College Healthcare NHS Trust

Robert Shulman
Lead Pharmacist, University College London Hospitals NHS Foundation Trust

Hugh Montgomery
Director, Centre for Human Health and Performance, University College London

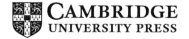

CAMBRIDGE
UNIVERSITY PRESS

University Printing House, Cambridge CB2 8BS, United Kingdom

One Liberty Plaza, 20th Floor, New York, NY 10006, USA

477 Williamstown Road, Port Melbourne, VIC 3207, Australia

314–321, 3rd Floor, Plot 3, Splendor Forum, Jasola District

Centre, New Delhi – 110025, India

79 Anson Road, #06-04/06, Singapore 079906

Cambridge University Press is part of the University of
Cambridge.

It furthers the University's mission by disseminating knowledge
in the pursuit of education, learning, and research at the highest
international levels of excellence.

www.cambridge.org
Information on this title: www.cambridge.org/9781108702478
DOI: 10.1017/9781108776936

© First edition published in 2007 by Remedica
© Cambridge University Press 2020

This publication is in copyright. Subject to statutory exception
and to the provisions of relevant collective licensing agreements,
no reproduction of any part may take place without the written
permission of Cambridge University Press.

First edition published 2007
Second edition published 2020

Printed in the United Kingdom by TJ International Ltd, Padstow
Cornwall

*A catalogue record for this publication is available from the British
Library.*

ISBN 978-1-108-70247-8 Paperback

Cambridge University Press has no responsibility for the persistence or accuracy of URLs for external or third-party internet websites referred to in this publication and does not guarantee that any content on such websites is, or will remain, accurate or appropriate.

Every effort has been made in preparing this book to provide accurate and up-to-date information that is in accord with accepted standards and practice at the time of publication. Although case histories are drawn from actual cases, every effort has been made to disguise the identities of the individuals involved. Nevertheless, the authors, editors, and publishers can make no warranties that the information contained herein is totally free from error, not least because clinical standards are constantly changing through research and regulation. The authors, editors and publishers therefore disclaim all liability for direct or consequential damages resulting from the use of material contained in this book. Readers are strongly advised to pay careful attention to information provided by the manufacturer of any drugs or equipment that they plan to use.

Contents

Contributors

Suparna Bali FFRPS MRPharmS
Principal Pharmacist – Surgical
    Services
Pharmacy Department
Royal Free London NHS Foundation
    Trust

**Samrina Bhatti MRPharmS
PGClinDip**
NHS Specialist Pharmacy Service
    and Centre for Medicines
    Optimisation Research and
    Education
University College London
    Hospitals NHS Foundation Trust

**Jim Bolton MB BS BSc (Hons)
FRCPsych**
Consultant Liaison Psychiatrist
St Helier Hospital, London
South West London & St George's
    Mental Health NHS Trust

**Alison Brown BPharm
PGClinDip**
Department of Haematological
    Medicine
King's Thrombosis Centre
King's College Hospital NHS
    Foundation Trust

**David Brull MBBS BSc MD
FRCP**
Consultant Cardiologist
Whittington Health NHS Trust,
    Barts Health NHS Trust

Rosalind Byrne BPharm PGClinDip
Lead Pharmacist Anticoagulation
Department of Haematological
    Medicine
King's Thrombosis Centre
King's College Hospital NHS
    Foundation Trust

Bridget Coleman
Deputy Chief Pharmacist,
    Whittington Health NHS Trust
Honorary Senior Lecturer,
    University College London

Miriam Conway
Diabetes Specialist Nurse
Independent Nurse Prescriber
Whittington Health NHS Trust

Laura Coughlan BSc RD
Gastroenterology Dietician
Whittington Health NHS Trust

**Nishma Gadher MPharm
PGDipGPP**
Senior Critical Care Pharmacist
University College London
    Hospitals NHS Foundation Trust

**Ned Gilbert-Kawai MBChB MSc
(Hons) PhD FRCA MRCP FRGS
DRCOG FHEA**
Anaesthesia and Intensive Care
    Medicine Specialist Registrar
Royal London Hospital, Barts
    Health NHS Trust

Xolani Dereck Gondongwe PhD
Lead Pharmacist – Education
University College London
  Hospitals NHS Foundation Trust

Alia Husain MRPharmS PGDipGPP
Senior Clinical Pharmacist for
  Women's Health and Neonates
University College London
  Hospitals NHS Foundation Trust

**Shirley Ip BPharm(Hons)
Independent Prescriber**
Lead Pharmacist, Care of Older
  People, Whittington Health NHS
  Trust
Lead Frailty Pharmacist,
  Hertfordshire and West Essex STP

Yogini Jani FFRPS, MRPharmS
Consultant Pharmacist & EHRS
  Patient Safety Lead
Director, UCLH-UCL Centre for
  Medicines Optimisation Research
  and Education
University College London
  Hospitals NHS Foundation Trust

Dipty Joshi BSc (Hons) MPharm IP
University College London

**Lloyd E. Kwanten FANZCA MRCA
MBBS (Hons) BMedSc (Hons)
GD-CLINUS**
Locum Consultant in
  Cardiothoracic Anaesthesia,
Lead for Quality Improvement for
  Perioperative Medicine
Department of Perioperative
  Medicine
Barts Heart Centre
Barts Health NHS Trust

**Roman Landowski MRPharmS
PGDip Clin Phcy**
University College London

**Katherine Le Bosquet MPharm
PGDip GPP IP MRPharmS**
Lead Pharmacist for Frailty and
  Elderly Medicine, Medway NHS
  Foundation Trust

**Hugh Montgomery MB BS BSc
FRCP MD FRGS FRSB FRI FFICM**
Professor of Intensive Care
  Medicine, University College
  London
Consultant Intensivist, Whittington
  Health NHS Trust

**Mayur Murali MB BS BSc (Hons)
MSc MRCP DTM&H FHEA**
Anaesthetic Registrar
Imperial College Healthcare NHS
  Trust

Simon Noble MD FRCP
Marie Curie Professor in Supportive
  and Palliative Medicine
Cardiff University

**Jessal Mitul Palan MBBS BSc
(Hons)**
MRCP Specialty Trainee in Diabetes &
  Endocrinology and General
  Medicine
University College London
  Hospitals NHS Foundation Trust

**Abimbola Sanu ClinDip
MRPharmS**
EHRS Senior Designer/Analyst –
  Pharmacy and Cancer
University College London
  Hospitals NHS Foundation Trust

Robert Shulman FFRPS FRPharmS
Lead Pharmacist – Critical Care
Pharmacy Department
University College London
Hospitals NHS Foundation
Trust

Angad Singh
Gastroenterology Specialist
Registrar
Whittington Health NHS Trust

Lindsey Stockford MPharm DipClinPharm
Senior Clinical Pharmacist
National Hospital for Neurology and
Neurosurgery
University College London
Hospitals NHS Foundation Trust

Sheetal Sumaria BSc (Pharm) DipClinPharm
Lead of Clinical Services
National Hospital for Neurology and
Neurosurgery
University College London
Hospitals NHS Foundation Trust

Sebastian Vandermolen MBBS MRCP
Cardiology Registrar
Barts Heart Centre
Barts Health NHS Trust

A Peter R Wilson MA MD FRCP FRCPath FFICM
Consultant Microbiologist
Clinical Microbiology & Virology
University College London
Hospitals NHS Foundation Trust

Preface to the Second Edition

Since the first edition of this book appeared, much has changed: most notably, prescribing nurse practitioners and prescribing pharmacists have appeared. But much has stayed the same: 'clinical pharmacology' textbooks still offer 'facts about drugs', and the (excellent) British National Formulary is especially helpful when 'one knows what one wants to know'. *Surviving Prescribing* fills a gap that remains, offering clear, precise and concise practical advice to all who prescribe. It is a 'wise and experienced senior', portable in the pocket. It has helped a generation of prescribers already. We hope that it will likewise help you.

Abbreviations

$5HT_3$	serotonin
ABG	arterial blood gas
ABW	actual body weight
ACE inhibitors/ACEi	angiotensin converting enzyme inhibitors
ACh	acetylcholine
ACS	acute coronary syndrome
AF	atrial fibrillation
AIDS	acquired immune deficiency syndrome
AKI	acute kidney injury
ALT	alanine aminotransferase
APTT	activated partial thromboplastin time
ARB	angiotensin II receptor blockers
AV	atrioventricular
BD	bis in die (twice a day)
BIPAP	bilevel positive airway pressure
BMI	body mass index
BNF	British National Formulary
BP	blood pressure
BPH	benign prostatic hyperplasia
bpm	beats per minute
Ca^{2+}	calcium
CBG	capillary blood glucose
CBW	corrected body weight
CCF	congestive cardiac failure
CDS	clinical decision support
CHA_2DS_2-VASc	scoring system to guide antithrombotic treatment in atrial fibrillation
CKD	chronic kidney disease
CNS	central nervous system
CO_2	carbon dioxide
COPD	chronic obstructive pulmonary disease
COX-2	cyclooxygenase-2
CPAP	continuous positive airway pressure
CrCl	creatinine clearance
CRF	chronic renal failure
CRP	C-reactive protein
CSF	cerebrospinal fluid
CT	computed tomography

CYP 3A/450	cytochrome P450 3A4
D_2	dopamine 2 receptor
DKA	diabetic ketoacidosis
DOAC	direct oral anticoagulant
DoLS	Deprivation of Liberty Safeguards
DPP-4 inhibitors	inhibitors of dipeptidyl peptidase-4
DTs	delirium tremens
DVT	deep vein thrombosis
ECG	electrocardiogram
ED	erectile dysfunction
EF	ejection fraction
eGFR	estimated glomerular filtration rate
EMR	endoscopic mucosal resection
ERCP	endoscopic retrograde cholangio-pancreatography
ESD	endoscopic submucosal dissection
EUS	endoscopic ultrasound
FBC	full blood count
FNA	fine needle aspiration
FRII	fixed-rate insulin infusion
FY2	Foundation Year 2
GCS	Glasgow Coma Score
GFR	glomerular filtration rate
GI	gastrointestinal
GLP-1 agonist	glucagon-like peptide-1 agonist
GP	general practitioner
GTN	glyceryl trinitrate
GU	genitourinary
H_2	histamine 2 receptor
HbA1c	haemoglobin A1c
HD	haemodialysis
HDU	high dependency unit
HHS	hyperosmolar hyperglycaemic state
HIV	human immunodeficiency virus
HP	high potency
HONC	hyperosmolar non-ketotic coma
HR	heart rate
HRT	hormone replacement therapy
IBD	inflammatory bowel disease
IBW	ideal body weight
ICP	intracranial pressure
ICU	intensive care unit
IM	intramuscular
INR	international normalised ratio
IPC	intermittent pneumatic compression

IU	international units
IV	intravenous
JBDS	Joint British Diabetes Societies
JVP	jugular venous pressure
K^+	potassium
KCl	potassium chloride
kg	kilograms
L	litre
LA	local anaesthetic
LFTs	liver function tests
LMWH	low molecular weight heparin
LP	lumbar puncture
LV	left ventricle
LVF	left ventricular failure
MAP	mean arterial pressure
mcg/µg	micrograms
MCV	mean corpuscular volume
MDT	multidisciplinary team
mg	milligrams
Mg^{2+}	magnesium
MHRA	Medicines and Healthcare products Regulatory Agency
MI	myocardial infarction
min	minute
mL	millilitres
mmHg	millimetres of mercury
mmol	millimoles
mosmol	milliosmoles
MR	modified release
MRA	magnetic resonance angiography
MRSA	methillin-resistant *Staphylococcus aureus*
MST	morphine slow-release tablet
Na^+	sodium
NAC	*N*-acetylcysteine
NaCl	sodium chloride
NBM	nil by mouth
NG	nasogastric
NH_3	ammonia
NH_4^+	ammonium
NICE	National Institute for Health and Care Excellence
nocte	at night
NSAID	non-steroidal anti-inflammatory drug
NSTEMI	non-ST-elevation MI
OD	omne in die (once daily)

OM	omni mane (every morning)
ON	omne nocte (every night)
PAH	pulmonary arterial hypertension
PCA	patient-controlled analgesia
PCC	prothrombin complex concentrate
PCI	percutaneous coronary intervention
PE	pulmonary embolism
PEFR	peak expiratory flow rate
PEG	percutaneous endoscopic gastrostomy
PN	parenteral nutrition
PO	per os (orally)
PO_4^{2-}	phosphate
PPI	proton pump inhibitor
PR	per rectum (rectally)
PRN	pro re nata (as needed)
PT	prothrombin time
PTH	parathyroid hormone
PTU	propylthiouracil
QDS	quarter die sumendum (four times daily)
QTc	corrected QT interval
RV	right ventricle
SA	sinoatrial
SAH	subarachnoid haemorrhage
SaO_2	arterial blood oxygen saturation
SBP	systolic blood pressure
SC	subcutaneous
SGLT2 inhibitors	sodium/glucose co-transporter 2 inhibitors
SIADH	syndrome of inappropriate ADH secretion
sPESI	simplified pulmonary embolism severity index
SSRI	selective serotonin reuptake inhibitor
STAT	statim (immediately)
STEMI	ST-elevation MI
SVT	supraventricular tachycardia
T3	triiodothyronine
T4	thyroxine
TB	tuberculosis
TDM	therapeutic drug monitoring
TDS	ter die sumendum (three times daily)
TED	thromboembolism deterrent
THR	total hip replacement
TKR	total knee replacement
TPN	total parenteral nutrition
TSH	thyroid stimulating hormone

U	units
VBG	venous blood gas
VF	ventricular fibrillation
VRII	variable-rate insulin infusion
VT	ventricular tachycardia
VTE	venous thromboembolism

Chapter 1
The Basics of Safe Drug Use
Yogini Jani

Here, 'safe drug use' refers to your prescription and administration, not recreational use. In this regard, there are a few 'golden rules' which will keep you out of trouble (and court!).

Ready?

You can't be expected to 'know it all' let alone remember it all. So seek references!

a. Find local policies/protocols in your hospital formulary and use them.

b. Check the BNF when in doubt. It is now available online and as an app too (https://bnf.nice.org.uk). Remember that, as well as dosing, it will tell you indications, contraindications, interactions, side effects, use in hepatic and renal failure, and use in pregnancy. It also includes National Institute of Health and Care Excellence (NICE) guidelines, other disease management guidelines (e.g. British Thoracic Guidelines on acute asthma), and an 'important safety advice section' that highlights warnings issued by the Commission on Human Medicines (CHM) or the Medicines and Healthcare products Regulatory Agency (MHRA).

c. Ask your pharmacy for help as a matter of routine, not just when 'it's all gone wrong'!

d. If the organisation is using electronic prescribing systems, many standard reference sources such as the BNF online, local protocols and national guidelines may be available as links: learn to use them effectively.

Steady…

Whether your hospital uses a paper chart (this is becoming rare but always good to know your way round one in case of technology failures!), or a funky electronic system, there will be separate prescribing sections. These include sections for one off 'STAT' doses of drugs, regular medications, as required 'PRN' drugs, infusions and intravenous fluids. There may also be supplementary charts or separate sections for 'specialist' items, e.g. total parenteral nutrition, anticoagulation and chemotherapy.

Beware

- ... of where you write/order your prescription! If incorrectly done, it may mean your patient does not get the drug, or you end up correcting lots of charts.
- In electronic systems, take care with default start times and dates – for once a day doses, the system may schedule the first dose for the next available time-slot – which may be too late for your patient.

GO!

You have now decided what to prescribe and at what dose, and have chosen which section to write/order the prescription. Now use 'SICKLy' tips to avoid mistakes:

Simplify. Try NOT to give drugs at all. All drugs have side effects and are hazardous. Every now and then, the drug you give will contribute (directly or indirectly) to a death. Did you know that the World Health Organization estimates an annual cost of $42 billion due to preventable medication harm?

Do you really have to give it? Will the green spit or sore throat not get better on its own? Is the cough so bad that codeine linctus and its side effects of constipation and drowsiness are worth it? Can you do anything that avoids drugs? e.g. reassurance, ear plugs if noise is keeping a patient awake, fruit and coffee for constipation?

Try to STOP (or 'deprescribe') a drug every time you review a chart.

Wherever possible, seek the 'once-a-day' drug from a class. Compliance will be better on discharge and the fewer the 'prescribing events' the fewer things that can go wrong!

Interrogate your patient and their charts: *Are all their allergies documented?* And what does the patient mean by 'allergy' to toxocillin? That they got a runny nose, or a rash or 'full blown' anaphylaxis? Were you just about to prescribe a drug that will make their skin peel off?

What is your patient's weight? You will need to know this to prescribe certain drugs, e.g. low molecular weight heparin, intravenous paracetamol and once daily gentamicin. Importantly, has the patient's weight changed significantly since the drug was prescribed, thus changing the prescribed dose?

What is your patient's height? This is needed to calculate surface area or ideal/excess body weight, which are required for gentamicin dosing and chemotherapeutics.

Clarify. Be clear in *writing/ordering* a prescription. Do not rush. Is there ANY chance that your script will be misread if on paper? Or that you may MIS-SELECT from an alphabetical electronic list of similar names?

Be clear in *reasoning*. Add comments where needed e.g. 'patient has been on sleepazepam for 20 years and withdraws without it: please give'.

Be clear with *timing*, in particular, start and stop times. We have all heard of patients still taking a loading dose of amiodarone daily, until their lungs are ruined with fibrosis. Clearly indicate on the chart when you want the course to be changed. Prescribe the 'reducing doses' for a full course, so that when you are next doing 'days' you don't still find the patient on 60 mg prednisolone 5 weeks on!

Check. Check *doses* etc. of unfamiliar drugs before prescribing. Electronic systems may highlight these as pop-up alerts. Resist the temptation to hit enter too quickly – make sure you READ what it says!

Check for *interactions* with the other charted drugs.

Check the doctor was correct in what they wrote, if you are *administering*.

Check everything you do at least twice. With intravenous drugs, NEVER be lazy. When tired, you can read what you expect to see. Ask someone else to check the ampoule or vial against the prescription ALWAYS!

Know. Have a basic understanding of the class of drug you are giving. Know a line or two about how it works. This is your safety lock: it allows you to hear alarm bells, nudging you to recall a drug interaction or side effect. Back this up revising from time to time the basic side effects and interactions of a drug and its class in a bigger textbook. If your patient does react, then manage them, but think about future treatment: is it an allergy (confirmed by testing) or an intolerance (side effect that may be managed in case of benefit/risk)? Document the reaction so that it can be communicated to the whole team and eventually the GP, and educate the patient about future implications.

Think Levels! Consider factors that might alter drug levels, e.g. age, disease, other drugs? Consider if the drug you are about to prescribe needs its levels monitored? Are you sure? *Check.* Call pharmacy. Call microbiology. Call a colleague. But *do call!* If yes, be clear about when levels should be taken, and how often. And ensure they are taken and acted upon. Put some fail safes in – mark the chart 'not to be given until Dr has reviewed levels' or 'do not give until INR has been seen'. On electronic systems, you can 'prescribe' the levels too, and the whizzier e-prescribing systems can be set up with rules so the dose cannot be given unless the result is available. And, lastly, think who will continue to review their levels when they are discharged? Have you booked them into anticoagulant clinic?

So, familiarise yourself with the chart and back yourself up with some information. Then, think:

SICKLy:

Simplify the chart (fewer drugs, fewer doses).

Interrogate the notes/charts/patient for contraindications, allergies and interactions. Take note of and act on electronic alerts.

Clarify your chart. Be clear with your writing/ordering, reasoning and timing.

Check doses, interactions and all ampoules or vials.

Know your drug classes, their mechanisms and major side effects/interactions.

Levels: think about factors that alter levels, and the need for monitoring them.

Finally, congratulations! Your patient has survived! Now safely DISCHARGE them!

1. Note the patient's discharge medications carefully, following the rules as above.

2. Mark clearly any changes from their admission medications, and include reasons for these changes.

3. Ensure the patient is aware of these changes: drugs will only work if the patient actually takes them – correctly.

4. Organise necessary follow-up, e.g. repeat phenytoin or INR levels, GP appointment after completion of steroid reduction for acute asthma etc.

Prescribing in Renal Disease
Dipty Joshi

Don't *cause* renal failure!

Kidneys are desperately sensitive to damage by drugs: fully 20% of acute kidney injury (AKI) episodes are drug-induced! Be afraid. Be *very* afraid. And then take care:

- Identify patients at risk and, if possible, eliminate these risk factors.
- Avoid potentially nephrotoxic agents wherever possible.
- Adjust drug doses, where necessary, in all those with pre-existing renal impairment, as drug accumulation and toxicity can quickly develop.

Many drugs are potentially nephrotoxic, and the list is too long to remember. However, high-risk *classes* to **AVOID** are as follows:

ACE Inhibitors and ARBs

ACE inhibitors and ARBs lower glomerular filtration pressure and can aid tubular uptake of other nephrotoxic drugs. Take care in patients with pre-existing renal disease, those who are dehydrated, those taking other potentially nephrotoxic drugs and those with possible renal artery stenosis. If worried, monitor blood pressure and biochemical markers of renal function carefully.

Iodinated Contrast Media/Dye

Risk is particularly high in patients with pre-existing renal impairment and in those with dehydration. In 50% of diabetics with impaired renal function, renal function declines further after use of radiocontrast agents. Hydration with a balanced salt solution (Hartmann's/Ringer's lactate) is a key preventative strategy. Hydration with sodium bicarbonate 1.26% can help in high-risk patients.

Antibiotics

Antibiotics can be directly tubulotoxic, or can cause allergic interstitial nephritis or crystallisation within the renal tubules. Aminoglycosides are a common

5

culprit: even with proper dose adjustment (see Chapter 37 – Therapeutic Drug Monitoring) there is no guarantee of safety and nephrotoxicity can still occur at therapeutic levels. Penicillins, cephalosporins and quinolones are also common culprits.

Lithium

Careful monitoring of levels is crucial.

NSAIDs and COX-2 Inhibitors

Risk rises with dose. If worried, think of alternatives (see Chapter 23 – Analgesia).

You should especially **AVOID** using such classes in combination: gentamicin + cephalosporin in the infected renal stone patient is bad enough but add diclofenac for the pain and …!

TOP TIPS to Avoid Drug Toxicity

- Don't exceed the recommended dose.
- For patients at risk of AKI, reduce the dose, concentration and/or rate of administration.
- Where necessary, monitor drug levels closely (e.g. vancomycin or gentamicin).
- Tailor the drug therapy to the individual needs of each patient with renal insufficiency. Some patients might still have some residual function left, which you will want to try to preserve for as long as possible.
- Periodic monitoring of renal function and urine output is particularly important in patients with renal impairment or at risk of developing AKI.

IF IN DOUBT, ASK YOUR HOSPITAL PHARMACIST!

Before choosing an appropriate drug and dosage schedule, the severity of renal impairment must be assessed. This is done by estimating the GFR.

Treatment of the Patient with Known Chronic Renal Impairment

Ok, so now the patient has presented with chronic renal failure (CRF). What drugs might they need? Here is a rough guide!

- Hypertension – a slight decrease in BP can have a significant effect in rescuing the patient's renal function. For example, ACE inhibitors can reduce the rate of loss of function, even if the blood pressure is normal but the protein:urea ratio is high.
- Oedema – treatment with high doses of loop diuretics (e.g. furosemide 250 mg–2 g/day ± metolazone 5–10 mg/day) might be required.

- Renal bone disease – give phosphate binders (e.g. sevelamer) and vitamin D analogues (alphacalcidol) and treat as soon as there is an increase in parathyroid hormone.
- Dietary advice – aim to restrict sodium intake as this will help to control BP and prevent oedema. Restrict potassium if there is evidence of hyperkalaemia and acidosis, in which case treat with bicarbonate supplements. Reduce dietary phosphate intake.
- Anaemia – treat with erythropoietin. Give iron if deficient.
- Hyperlipidaemia – this will increase the risk of cardiovascular disease and contribute to renal insufficiency. Use statins as first line.

Do your sums!

Drug doses can be adjusted according to the patient's estimated (or measured) creatinine clearance (CrCl). The most accurate method of determining CrCl is to gather urine over 24 hours, and then use the following equation:

$$CrCl = UV / Pt$$

where:

U = urinary creatinine concentration (mmol/L)

V = volume of urine (mL)

P = plasma creatinine concentration (mmol/L)

t = time (minutes)

A quicker and less cumbersome method that is widely used to measure the adult plasma creatinine concentration (and hence renal function) is with the Cockroft and Gault equation:

$$CrCl = \frac{G \times (140 - age\ in\ years) \times weight\ in\ kg}{serum\ creatinine\ (mmol/L)}$$

where:

G = 1.04 (females) or 1.23 (males)

Height and body weight are critically important to calculate drug dosages – particularly in obese or oedematous patients, use ideal body weight.

A point to remember about the Crockroft and Gault equation is that it merely provides an approximation of creatinine clearance, particularly when the clinical setting is dynamic and the renal function might be changing on a daily basis. The equation is useful when renal dysfunction is stable. However, in AKI, creatinine concentrations might not have reached steady state and so might not reflect the true functional capacity of the kidneys.

As a broad classification, renal impairment is divided into three groups for prescribing purposes (Table 2.1).

Table 2.1 Renal impairment classification groups

Grade	GFR (mL/min)	Serum creatinine (mmol/L)
Mild	20–50	150–300
Moderate	10–20	300–700
Severe	<10	>700

Armed with this classification, you are now in position to choose the right dose from the Table 2.2.

Table 2.2 Drug doses in renal impairment

Drug	CrCl (mL/minutes)	Dose
Aciclovir PO	20–50	Normal
	10–20	Herpes simplex: 200 mg QDS to TDS
		Herpes zoster: 400–800 mg TDS
	<10	Herpes simplex: 200 mg BD
		Herpes zoster: 400–800 mg BD
Aciclovir IV	25–50	5–10 mg/kg BD
	10–25	5–10 mg/kg BD
	<10	2.5–5 mg/kg BD
Allopurinol	20–50	200–300 mg OD
	10–20	100–200 mg OD
	<10	100 mg OD/alternate day
Amikacin IV	20–50	5–6 mg/kg BD
	10–20	3–4 mg/kg BD
	<10	2 mg/kg every 24–48 hours
Amoxicillin PO/IV	20–50	Dose as per normal renal function
	10–20	Dose as per normal renal function
	<10	250 mg TDS
Amphotericin IV	<50	Seek advice
Anakinra	30–50	Dose as per normal renal function
	10–30	100 mg on alternate days
	<10	100 mg on alternate days
Apixaban	30–50	Dose as per normal renal function. Use with caution
	15–30	AF: 2.5 mg twice daily
		Use with caution
	<15	Manufacturers advise to avoid

Drug	CrCl (mL/minutes)	Dose
Avanafil	30–50	Dose as per normal renal function
	10–30	Use with caution
	<10	Use with caution
Azathioprine	20–50	Dose as per normal renal function
	10–20	75–100%
	<10	50–75%
Benzylpenicillin IV	20–50	Dose as per normal renal function
	10–20	75%
	<10	20–50%
Bisoprolol	20–50	Dose as per normal renal function
	10–20	Dose as per normal renal function
	<10	1.25–10 mg OD
Cariprazine	30–50	Dose as per normal renal function
	<30	Cariprazine has not been evaluated in patients with severe (CrCl < 30 mL/min) renal impairment
Cefotaxime IV	20–50	Dose as per normal renal function
	10–20	Dose as per normal renal function
	<10	Load with 1 g then BD dose at same frequency
Ceftazidime IV	31–50	1 g BD[a]
	16–30	1 g OD[a]
	6–15	500 mg–1 g OD[a]
	<5	500 mg–1 g 48-hourly[a]
Ceftriaxone IV	10–50	Dose as per normal renal function
	<10	Use with caution in patients with severe renal impairment as well as hepatic insufficiency. In severe infection, dose at 1 g OD and increase to 2 g if necessary.
Cefuroxime IV	20–50	750 mg–1.5 g TDS
	10–20	750 mg–1.5 g TDS to BD
	<10	1.5 g OD
Chloral hydrate	20–50	Dose as per normal renal function
	10–20	500 mg nocte
	<10	Avoid
Ciprofloxacin	20–50	Dose as per normal renal function
	10–20	50% of normal dose
	<10	50% of normal dose

(cont.)

Table 2.2 *(cont.)*

Drug	CrCl (mL/minutes)	Dose
Clarithromycin	20–50	Dose as per normal renal function
	10–20	PO: 250–500 mg BD to OD
		IV: 250–500 mg BD
	<10	PO: 250 mg BD to OD
		IV: 250 mg BD
Clevidipine	10–50	Dose as per normal renal function
Clindamycin	10–50	Dose as per normal renal function
Clonidine	10–50	Dose as per normal renal function
Co-amoxiclav	30–50	Dose as per normal renal function
	10–30	PO: Dose as per normal renal function
		IV: 1.2 g BD
	<10	PO: 375 mg TDS
		IV: 1.2 g STAT followed by 600 mg to 1.2 g OD
Co-codamol/	20–50	Dose as per normal renal function
Co-dydramol	10–20	75–100% of normal dose
Co-trimoxazole PO/IV	>25	Dose as per normal renal function
	25–15	Normal dose for 3 days, then half standard dose
	<15	To be given if haemodialysis facilities are available. Normal dose for 3 days than half standard dose
Colchicine	20–50	Reduce dose or increase dosage interval by 50%.
	10–20	Reduce dose or increase dosage interval by 50%.
	<10	500 mcg 3–4 times a day; maximum total dose of 3 mg
Dabigatran	30–50	VTE prophylaxis: 75 mg within 1–4 hours of completed surgery and thereafter 150 mg once daily; 75 mg if also on CYP450 inhibitor
		AF/DVT/PE: 110–150 mg twice daily
	<10–30	Contraindicated
Dapagliflozin	20–50	Avoid
Degarelix	20–50	Dose as per normal renal function
	<10	Dose as per normal renal function. Use with caution
Doxazosin	<50	Dose as per normal renal function
Doxycyline	<50	Dose as per normal renal function
Dulaglutide	10–50	Dose as per normal renal function
Dutasteride	10–50	Dose as per normal renal function

Drug	CrCl (mL/minutes)	Dose
Edoxaban	15–50	30 mg once daily
	<15	Manufacturers advise to avoid
Enalapril	20–50	Dose as per normal renal function
	10–20	Start with 2.5 mg/day then dose to response
	<10	Start with 2.5 mg/day then dose to response
Erythromycin	20–50	Dose as per normal renal function
	10–20	Dose as per normal renal function
	<10	50–75% of normal dose, maximum 1.5 g/day
Ethambutol	20–50	Dose as per normal renal function
	10–20	Normal dose 24- to 36-hourly
	<10	Normal dose 48-hourly
Everolimus	20–50	Dose as per normal renal function
	10–20	Dose as per normal renal function
	<10	Dose as per normal renal function
Evolocumab	30–50	Dose as per normal renal function
	<10–30	Dose as per normal renal function. Use with caution
Flucloxacillin	10–50	Dose as per normal renal function
	<10–20	Dose as per normal renal function
Fluconazole	20–50	Dose as per normal renal function
	10–20	Dose as per normal renal function
	<10	50% of normal dose
Foscarnet IV	<50	See local guidelines
Gabapentin	60–90	400 mg TDS
	30–60	300 mg BD
	15–30	300 mg OD
	<15	300 mg 48-hourly
Ganciclovir IV	>70	5 mg/kg BD
	50–69	2.5 mg/kg BD
	25–49	2.5 mg/kg OD
	10–24	1.25 mg/kg OD
	<10	1.25 mg/kg OD
Gentamicin	<50	See local guidelines
Haloperidol	20–50	Dose as per normal renal function
	10–20	Dose as per normal renal function
	<10	Start with lower dose. Will accumulate
Heparin	30–50	Dose as per normal renal function
	<30	50% normal dose

(cont.)

Table 2.2 *(cont.)*

Drug	CrCl (mL/minutes)	Dose
Hydroxyurea	20–50	100% of normal dose
	10–20	50% of normal dose and titrate to response
	<10	20% of normal dose and titrate to response
Imipenem	50–30	500 mg QDS to TDS
	30–20	500 mg TDS to BD
	20–10	250–500 mg BD
	<10	250 mg BD
Isosorbide di/ mononitrate	<50	Dose as per normal renal function
Itraconazole	<50	Dose as per normal renal function
Labetalol	<50	Dose as per normal renal function
Lansoprazole	<50	Dose as per normal renal function
Linezolid PO/IV	<50	Dose as per normal renal function
Lomitapide	15–50	Dose as per normal renal function
	<15	Maximum dose 40 mg daily
Meloxicam	20–50	Dose as per normal renal function
	10–20	Dose as per normal renal function but avoid if possible.
	<10	Dose as per normal renal function but avoid if possible. Only use if on dialysis
Meropenem	20–50	500 mg–1 g BD
	10–20	250 mg–1 g BD or 500 mg TDS
	<10	250 mg–1 g OD
Metformin	30–50	25–50% of dose
	10–30	Contraindicated
	<10	Contraindicated
Methyldopa	20–50	250–500 mg TDS
	10–20	250–500 mg BD to TDS
	<10	250–500 mg OD to BD
Mirabegron	30–60	Dose as per normal renal function. 25 mg with CYP 3A inhibitors
	15–30	25 mg daily. Avoid with CYP 3A inhibitors
	<15	25 mg daily. Avoid with CYP 3A inhibitors
Morphine	20–50	75% of normal
	10–20	Use small doses, e.g. 2.5–5 mg
	<10	Use small doses, e.g. 1.25–2.5 mg
Nintedanib	30–50	Dose as per normal renal function
	<10–30	Dose as per normal renal function. Use with caution

Drug	CrCl (mL/minutes)	Dose
Oxycodone	20–50	Start with 75% of dose. Dose as per normal renal function
	10–20	Start with 75% of dose. Dose as per normal renal function
	<10	Start with small doses, e.g. 50% of dose
Oxytetracycline	20–50	Dose as per normal renal function
	10–20	0.5–1 g OD
	<10	0.5–1 g every 48-hourly
Penicillin V	<50	Dose as per normal renal function
Phenytoin	<50	Dose as per normal renal function
Pregabalin	20–50	Initial dose 75 mg daily and titrate according to tolerability and response
	10–20	Initial dose 25–50 mg daily and titrate according to tolerability and response
	<10	Initial dose 25 mg daily and titrate according to tolerability and response
Pyrazinamide	50–10	Dose as per normal renal function
	<10	Reduce size or frequency of dose
Rifampicin	50–10	Dose as per normal renal function
	<10	50–100% of normal dose
Rivaroxaban	30–50	AF: 15 mg once daily. DVT/PE: 15 mg twice daily for 3 weeks then 15–20 mg once daily
	15–29	Use with caution. AF: 15 mg once daily. DVT/PE: 15 mg twice daily for 3 weeks then 15–20 mg once daily
	<15	Contraindicated
Sodium fusidate	<50	Dose as per normal renal function
Sodium valproate	<50	Dose as per normal renal function
Sotalol	20–50	50% of normal dose
	10–20	25% of normal dose
	<10	Avoid
Streptomycin	<50	Reduce dose and measure levels
Tadalafil	20–50	ED: 5–10 mg not more than every 48 hours. BPH: 2.5–5 mg daily; PAH: 20–40 mg daily
	10–20	ED: 5–10 mg not more than every 72 hours and use with caution. BPH/PAH: Avoid
	<10	ED: 5–10 mg not more than every 72 hours and use with caution. BPH/PAH: Avoid
Tamoxifen	<50	Dose as per normal renal function

(cont.)

Table 2.2 (cont.)

Drug	CrCl (mL/minutes)	Dose
Tazocin	20–50	Dose as per normal renal function
	10–20	4.5 g BD
	<10	4.5 g BD
Teicoplanin	30–80	Normal dose for first 3 days then reduce: Give standard dose on alternate days
	<30 or HD	Give standard dose every third day
Thyroxine	<50	Dose as per normal renal function
Tramadol	20–50	Dose as per normal renal function
	10–20	50–100 mg BD
	<10	50 mg BD
Tranexamic acid	20–50	IV: 10 mg/kg 12 hourly
		PO: 25 mg/kg 12 hourly
	10–20	IV: 10 mg/kg 24 hourly
		PO: 25 mg/kg 12–24 hourly
	<10	IV: 5 mg/kg 24 hourly
		PO: 12.5 mg/kg 24 hourly
Trazodone	20–50	Dose as per normal renal function
	10–20	Dose as per normal renal function. Start with small doses and increase gradually
	<10	Start with small doses and increase gradually
Trimethoprim	>25	Dose as per normal renal function
	25–15	Normal dose for 3 days then half normal dose 18-hourly
	<15	Half normal dose OD
Urokinase	<50	Dose as per normal renal function
Valaciclovir	30–50	Dose as per normal renal function
	15–30	Herpes simplex: Dose as per normal renal function
		Herpes zoster: 1 g BD to OD
	<15	Herpes simplex: 500 mg OD
		Herpes zoster: 500 mg–1 g OD
Valganciclovir	40–59	Induction/treatment: 450 mg BD
		Maintenance/prophylaxis: 450 mg OD
	25–39	Induction/treatment: 450 mg OD
		Maintenance/prophylaxis: 450 mg 48-hourly
	10–24	Induction/treatment: 450 mg 48-hourly
		Maintainance/prophylaxis: 450 mg twice weekly
	<10	Treatment: 450 mg twice weekly

Drug	CrCl (mL/minutes)	Dose
Vancomycin	20–50	1 g STAT and adjust according to levels
	<20	1 g STAT and monitor serum levels at 24-hourly intervals
Venlafaxine	30–50	Dose as per normal renal function
	10–30	Reduce dose by 50% and administer OD
	<10	Reduce dose by 50% and administer OD
Vigabatrin	20–50	Give 50% of normal dose and titrate to response
	10–20	Give 25% of normal dose and titrate to response
	<10	Give 25% of normal dose and titrate to response
Warfarin	<50	Dose as per normal renal function
Zopiclone	10–50	Dose as per normal renal function
	<10	50 to 100% of normal dose

[a]Increase dose by 50% in severe infection.

Prescribing for Children

Abimbola Sanu

Definitions of Age Groups	
Neonate:	birth to 28 days (1 month)
Infant:	1 month to 2 years
Child:	2–12 years
Adolescent:	12–18 years

Myth Busters

- When it comes to prescribing, children are not 'little adults'.
- There is no such thing as a 'paediatric dose'! The dose and frequencies of medicines can change throughout childhood – and even in adolescents, standard adult doses are not always appropriate.

General Principles of Prescribing in Children

- Some adult drugs are unsuitable for use in children.
- Drug doses often don't just 'scale down' by weight.
- Fluid management in paediatric patients can be very complex – take extra care and don't be tempted to simply start fluids or continue them without appropriate supervision.
- Many products contain excipients that are risky for kids, e.g. alcohol (phenobarbital, ranitidine, senna), propylene glycol (pyridoxine injection) or dyes.

- Some sweetening agents have their own problems: large amounts of sorbitol cause diarrhoea, while aspartame contains phenylalanine, so must be used with caution in patients with phenylketonuria.

In addition, many drugs prescribed in children are 'off label' or unlicensed, for a variety of reasons (see box below). You can prescribe them, as long as you have taken the responsibility to personally ensure that you have adequate information to support the quality, efficacy, safety and use of the drug prior to prescribing. If you're not sure, ask. Don't leave it until the last minute.

Examples of Why a Drug Might be Unlicensed

- Manufactured under a special manufacturing licence
- Prepared extemporaneously
- Imported from another country
- Only just undergoing clinical trials in adults
- Product is not a medicine but is being used to treat a rare condition.

The best advice, therefore, is that unless you are a paediatrician you should not be prescribing! If you have to prescribe, always use a reputable paediatric formulary (e.g. BNF for children) and/or locally agreed policies – and then consult with a paediatrician if you have any doubt at all. The basic principles are no different to those in adults (see Chapter 1 – The Basics of Safe Drug Use). However, given that this might be unfamiliar ground – and that incorrect dosing can be catastrophic – remember the following to avoid medication errors.

TOP TIPS for Avoiding Medication Errors

- Always take care with calculations.
- Get an independent, second check if unsure.
- Write units out in full (e.g. micrograms NOT mcg or mg and units NOT U or IU).
- Never use a trailing zero (e.g. 5 mg NOT 5.0 mg).

Routes of Administration in Children

Table 3.1 Advantages and disadvantages of different routes of administration in children

Route	Advantages	Disadvantages
Intravenous	Predictable blood levels	Fragility of veins Risk of extravasation
Intramuscular	None	Painful Erratic absorption
Oral	Easiest Convenient Accurate administration with oral syringes	Lack of suitable dosage forms Mixing with feeds
Rectal	Rapid onset of action e.g. diazepam for fitting	Lack of suitable dosage forms Erratically absorbed e.g. theophylline
Inhalation	Spacers can improve delivery of drug Paediatric formularies will recommend suitable ones	Lack of coordination in young children

Adherence in Children

There's no point writing a prescription for a medicine the patient can't or won't take. Sometimes a tablet will be more manageable than three tablespoons of liquid that smells like cat pee! Involve parents/carers and, if possible, the child from a very early stage.

Both verbal and written information should be provided at a level that is easy to understand. Patient information leaflets provided by manufacturers can be helpful but will often state that products are 'not suitable for use in children', causing parents additional alarm and confusion. www.medicinesforchildren.org.uk is a resource which provides patient information leaflets tailored to paediatric use and concerns. Get your paediatric pharmacist involved in explaining the issues. They will also be able to help advise on different dosage forms and what to do if a tablet or capsule has to be manipulated.

TOP TIPS for Improving Compliance in Children

- Consider ease of administration
- Tailor to the child's daily routine
- Set treatment goals in collaboration with the child (if possible)
- Provide suitable information to caregivers.

Common Mistakes!

Avoid the following common problems:

- Think dose!

  Example: ALWAYS prescribe the DOSE, not the volume: e.g. 'furosemide 5 mL TDS' is a dangerous prescription! Formulations available are 1 mg/mL, 4 mg/mL, 8 mg/mL and 10 mg/mL – so the dose could vary each time … and overdose is possible.

- Think decimals!

  Example: morphine 2.0–4.0 mg could easily be read as 20–40 mg, rather than 2–4 mg … and can kill.

- Think 'non-adult' dose!

  Example: prescribing 1.5 g paracetamol for a large child on a dose/kg basis, rather than a ceiling of 1 g, is clearly wrong. It can cause liver failure and death.

Reporting Adverse Drug Reactions

Little is known about the safe use of some medicines in children. Children are not usually exposed to medicines in clinical trials. Be alert and report suspected adverse reactions. Never underestimate your role in this. Reports should be filled in on the usual Yellow Card system online. The MHRA has a subgroup that specifically focuses on paediatric medicines.

Prescribing for Older Patients

Shirley Ip

Who are Older Patients?

Older patients, especially if debilitated, deserve special thought when prescribing. We have to be careful about quantifying age with respect to 'older people'; however, 75-years plus is a good working definition, although many 65-year olds will appear to be physiologically older if they have had poor control of long-term conditions. So perhaps, the chronological age of the patient is not as important as the physiological age. Patient frailty also needs to be considered.

Special Considerations for Prescribing in Older Patients

As people become older, their care becomes fragmented; more and more things start to go wrong and these are often treated in isolation with no thought given to how these treatments work (or don't work!) together. Therefore, it is important to think holistically about the whole person when any treatment is initiated.

It is also useful to think about the wider context of any prescribed medication. Most drug trials will not have been conducted on older patients, so the outcomes seen in younger adults may not be replicable. Beware of the treatment outcomes; in younger patients, you may want to treat aggressively to achieve (for example) a low target blood pressure or blood sugar. In older patients, these aggressive treatment targets may not be wise, as low blood pressures and low blood sugars may run an increased risk of falls and result in major injuries such as fractured hips that can have devastating consequences.

Frailty

As individuals age, frailty becomes an increasing concern for the prescriber. Frailty is a loss of resilience so patients are unable to bounce back after a physical or mental illness, an accident or other stressful event. People living with frailty are likely to have several issues, which, taken individually, might not be very serious but when added together have a large impact on health, confidence

---

With acknowledgement to Anthony Grosso, who was the original author of this chapter.

and well-being. Individuals presenting with frailty are much more susceptible to drug/drug interactions and adverse drug reactions and therefore the prescriber must proceed with caution.

Cognitive Impairment in the Older Patient

Since 2016, dementia has overtaken cardiac disease as the biggest killer in the UK. In addition, stroke and psychiatric conditions can cause cognitive impairment. Therefore, prescribing for older people must give due consideration to a patient's mental capacity.

During episodes of acute illness, an older patient with no known cognitive impairment may experience episodes of acute delirium (see Chapter 7 – Management of the Delirious Patient), which needs to be managed in addition to their physical illness.

If you do not think that a patient has the capacity to make decisions around their care, ensure that the appropriate legal and ethical guidance is consulted, such as the Mental Health Act, the Mental Capacity Acts and the Deprivation of Liberty Safeguards (DoLS).

Decline in Organ Function with Age

Renal clearance capacity falls with age, meaning that older patients will eliminate some drugs and their metabolites more slowly than younger patients. Therefore, some drug doses should be reduced in older people. Further clearance can be reduced by acute illness or dehydration causing acute kidney injury (AKI) – so adverse or toxic effects might suddenly appear in a patient on a previously stable (and safe) dose. Older people are often more sensitive to adverse effects and some drugs are best avoided altogether. Meanwhile, the absorption, distribution and metabolism of some drugs is altered in older patients. You *must* therefore consult relevant references if in any doubt. Note that while the BNF may have an overview of some drugs when renal function is impaired, more complete advice should be sought from Chapter 2 of this book, specialist sources such as your pharmacist or the Renal Drug Database (see https://renaldrugdatabase.com/).

The eGFR (estimated glomerular filtration rate) should be used with caution. It often overestimates renal clearance. A more accurate calculation can be obtained from the equations in Chapter 2, or your friendly pharmacist.

Medication Adherence

Physical Barriers to Medication Adherence

As patients become older, with the increasing burden of multiple illness, they may develop physical barriers to adherence. As a prescriber, you should cater for these. Some examples are given below:

- Visual impairment: large print labels
- Poor dexterity: non-child proof lids
- Poor swallow: liquids
- Inability to administer medicines: training of informal carers or relatives/referral to district nurses
- Patient information leaflets/reminder charts to aid patients in taking multiple medications

Polypharmacy

Polypharmacy is a term that describes the use of many medicines in one individual. There may be perfectly valid reasons why a patient is prescribed many medicines, including having multiple chronic medical conditions. Often, though, inappropriate or problematic polypharmacy occurs, where more medicines than are needed continue to be prescribed. Medicines that continue to be prescribed when not required, or when impacting negatively on the individual's health and well-being, should be reviewed with a view to discontinuing or adjusting to minimise their negative impact (see Chapter 41 – Deprescribing).

When prescribing anything new, always think about what the patient is already taking, and how the new medication fits into the patient's current regimen.

Any rationalisation of medication regimens should be carried out with the aid of experienced prescribers/pharmacists with specialist knowledge of the use of medicines in older people, as stopping or adjusting one or more medications can have unintended adverse consequences, and additional monitoring may be required.

Shared Decision-Making in Prescribing Leading to Increased Adherence

When making changes to a patient's medication regimen, always consider what the patient, their relatives and their carers want as outcomes of their treatment. Always think about how you can involve your patient in shared decision-making about their treatment – this way, you can understand what the patient's priorities are, and you can be more assured that they will be adherent to prescribed medication.

For instance, a respiratory patient may not be interested in taking medication to improve their lung function tests but may be more likely to take them if they extend the distance they can walk so they can get to the local shop. Framing outcomes in the patients' terms can improve adherence.

Thinking About the Future

Always prescribe in relation to the whole patient and think about the future, i.e.:

- What are the treatment priorities and what are the treatment goals?
- How does the new treatment fit into their current medication regimen?
- Does the new medication impact on current care? e.g. New medication is given three times a day, but the patient only gets twice a day package of care and requires medication prompting. Can the new medication be adjusted?

Think about the risks versus the benefits of any treatments – for example anticoagulants in recurrent fallers.

Thought should be given to a patient's advance care plan or end of life care plan – for instance there is no need to continue drugs that will benefit a patient in years to come due to risk reduction, if the patient is nearing the end of life.

Prescribing in Pregnancy

Alia Husain

The thalidomide disaster of 1958 and later isotretinoin from 1995 showed that drugs *do* reach the fetus and can cause harm. Even now, of the 2–3% of babies born in the UK with a recognised birth defect, drugs (illicit or prescription) are implicated in 1–2%.

Think Before Prescribing!

There is often now a general perception that the use of any medication at any time in pregnancy could cause harm to the growing baby – but this is also not always the case!

Weighing the Risks

There are about 20 groups of medicines that are considered safe. A further similar number are recognised as having an increased risk to the fetus. However, for the majority there is no proof of safety or danger. Often, the advice of manufacturers is not to prescribe in pregnancy unless the benefit outweighs the risk. But in clinical practice what can you do to help make a safe decision?

Think of the Possible *Benefit* to the Mother

- Consider the danger of the condition. Are we talking threadworms or thrombosis, heart attack or heartburn? In other words, what is the risk of *not* treating?
- How effective is the drug likely to be? If the condition is not dangerous and the benefits of treatment are minor, are there any non-drug measures that might help, e.g. improved hygiene for 6 weeks to break a threadworm lifecycle? Milk for heartburn?
- Are there risks to the fetus from not treating the disease? This is the conundrum that you face when an epileptic tells you that she is

With acknowledgement to Roman Landowski, who was the original author of this chapter.

pregnant – both the disease and the treatments are known to have adverse effects on the fetus. In this case it is important to remember you are not alone and there are often specialist teams such as neurologists who can provide specialist advice.

Then, Think of the *Risk* to the Fetus

Most of the time, you don't know the risk to the fetus. But you do know that the risk is likely to change with the trimester. Drugs can be safe in one trimester and dangerous in another.

Pre-Embryonic Period

Drugs taken in the first 17 days after conception exert an 'all or nothing' effect. The cluster of cells is either completely killed off, which results in a late menstrual bleed and the woman most likely never realises she was pregnant, or the cells recover completely and develop normally. If exposure is confined to this period and the woman finds herself still pregnant then you can be more confident that drug has had no effect on the fetus.

First Trimester

The period of organ formation. This period holds the greatest risk of drug-induced teratogenesis, e.g. spina bifida is caused by antifolate medicine (methotrexate or trimethoprim) exposure at this time. Try to delay all non-urgent medications until the second trimester.

Second and Third Trimesters

The organs are developing and maturing. Drugs will affect their function rather than their structure, e.g. enalapril can cause fetal renal failure if exposure occurs at this time.

Exposure near term risks labour, perinatal and neonatal complications. Neonatal respiratory depression is a feature of pethidine administration during labour. But again, this doesn't mean that you cannot use pethidine for a mother in labour.

Then, Think *Form* of Administration

Topical drugs penetrate the placenta less – so reach for the topical clotrimazole rather than oral fluconazole when treating thrush.

- Check written sources
- Check with your registrar
- Check with your pharmacist.

In the BNF, each medicine monograph has basic information regarding its use in pregnancy; however, it may often lack detail and may cause uncertainty.

If you are not sure, don't take a chance; call your hospital pharmacist or local medicines information department.

Common Prescriptions

Analgesics

- Paracetamol is safe in all stages of pregnancy.
- Opiates like dihydrocodeine, morphine or methadone do not cause birth defects. However, if they are used throughout pregnancy then the neonate can experience a distressing withdrawal syndrome. Due to the risk of seizures, this is best managed on a neonatal unit.
- NSAIDs like ibuprofen or diclofenac can cause premature closure of the ductus arteriosus (leading to pulmonary hypertension) if used in late pregnancy. They can also cause an increase in maternal blood loss during labour due to their antiplatelet effects. There are, of course, certain conditions where NSAIDs might be prescribed in pregnancy (e.g. sulindac for polyhydramnios [excess amniotic fluid in the amniotic sac]).

Antiasthmatics

- Inhaled medicines are safe as they don't achieve significant blood levels. This includes salbutamol, which, when given systemically, relaxes the uterine muscle but when inhaled does not prolong labour.
- Systemic steroids (e.g. prednisolone) can increase the risk of cleft lip and cleft palate if used in the first trimester, so keep courses short. High-dose inhaled steroids (e.g. 1500 micrograms/day beclametasone) could theoretically carry the same risk. However, you may see systemic steroids being used for women with threatened preterm labour to help develop a baby's lungs.

Antibiotics

- Penicillins (e.g. amoxicillin, flucloxacillin) and cephalosporins (e.g. cefuroxime, cefalexin) are considered safe.
- Quinolones such as ciprofloxacin have caused fetal arthropathy in animal studies, but very rarely in humans. Nevertheless, they should be avoided where possible.
- Trimethoprim is an antifolate drug that has been associated with an increase in birth defects following first trimester exposure.
- Tetracyclines (e.g. doxycycline, oxytetracycline) cause permanent yellow–brown bands to appear on the teeth following exposure from about 24 weeks' gestation.

Anticoagulants

- Low molecular weight heparins are the safest as they do not cross the placenta. Some (e.g. dalteparin) have positive evidence for safety in pregnancy.
- Unfractionated heparin is safe for the fetus but can cause maternal osteoporosis if used for more than 6 months in pregnancy.
- Aspirin possibly increases the risk of abruptio placentae and stillbirth.
- Warfarin has been associated with fetal intracranial bleeds when used in the second and third trimesters, which might lead to in utero death. Fetal warfarin syndrome has also been described following exposure between gestational weeks 6–9. This includes nasal, ocular, ear, cardiac, skeletal and mental defects.

Antiemetics

- Antihistamines such as cyclizine and promethazine are the drugs of choice. They've been around for ages without evidence of harm.
- Ondansetron should not be used as first line in the treatment of nausea and vomiting in pregnancy. There is a possible link between ondansetron use in early pregnancy and cleft lip and/or palate in the baby, although current research suggests that the chance of this occurring is very small. It should be reserved for use after other agents have not worked.
- Prochlorperazine is also considered safe for the fetus, but young women are at increased risk of experiencing dose-related extrapyramidal side effects from it.

Anticonvulsants

In 2016 there was an MHRA alert that sodium valproate should not be used in any women who are pregnant or planning on becoming pregnant unless all other antiepileptic agents do not work. Of babies with mothers taking sodium valproate, 10% had a birth defect and 40% grew up with developmental problems.

Carbamazepine is associated with neural tube defects (e.g. spina bifida, anencephaly) when given in the first trimester. To counter this, folic acid 5 mg/day is co-prescribed throughout pregnancy. Carbamazepine, phenytoin and phenobarbital all induce the metabolism of vitamin K, so it is common to co-prescribe vitamin K for the last month of pregnancy to reduce the chance of vitamin K deficiency bleeding in the newborn.

Fetal antiepileptic syndrome refers to a range of somatic defects associated with the drugs mentioned. It includes cleft lip, cleft palate, hypertelorism, low-set ears, retrognathia and shortened distal phalanges. There is also some evidence that these drugs slow mental development in childhood, while a withdrawal reaction (agitation) has been seen in neonates exposed to phenobarbital and benzodiazepines such as clonazepam. The risks of defects can be lowered by reducing the number of antiepileptic drugs and the doses used to the minimum level where a mother has no seizures.

Antifungals

There is sufficient experience with clotrimazole cream and pessaries to assume that it is safe.

In the first trimester, avoid oral fluconazole as high doses ($\geq$400 mg) have been associated with craniofacial and skeletal defects similar to Antley–Bixler syndrome.

Antihypertensives

- Methyldopa and hydralazine are considered to be safe, mainly because they have been around for a long time without any obvious problems cropping up.
- Beta-blockers are associated with fetal growth restriction due to placental vasoconstriction, although this is less likely with the vasodilatory labetalol. This effect is most noticeable after exposure in the second and third trimesters. Beta-blockers at term can also cause neonatal bradycardia and hypoglycaemia (by increasing neonatal insulin and reducing glucagon).
- ACE inhibitors are known to reduce fetal renal function when prescribed in the second and third trimesters. Oligohydramnios ensues, which can lead to pulmonary hypoplasia and skeletal defects.
- ARBs (e.g. losartan, irbesartan) have similar pharmacological effects to ACE inhibitors, and so are assumed to carry similar risks.

Gastroprotective Agents

- There are reasonable data to assume that ranitidine and omeprazole are generally safe in pregnancy.
- Misoprostol is a uterine stimulant that causes uterine contractions; it can be found in combination with diclofenac. There is a risk of miscarriage if it is used at any stage of pregnancy.

Laxatives

- Senna is licensed, so is as safe as drugs in pregnancy get.
- Glycerin suppositories, lactulose and ispaghula work locally and have minimal systemic absorption, and so are also safe.

Psychiatric Drugs

- Tricyclic antidepressants (e.g. amitriptyline, lofepramine) and SSRIs (e.g. fluoxetine, citalopram, sertraline) are not associated with birth defects, although they might cause an increased risk of miscarriage.

Neonatal withdrawal syndrome (insomnia, crying, poor feeding) are possible in infants exposed in utero in the last few months of pregnancy. This is particularly an issue with paroxetine, where cases of hypoglycaemia have also been seen.

- Lithium increases the risk of Ebstein's anomaly (inferior displacement of the tricuspid valve leaflets), but the absolute incidence in such infants is still very low (probably <1%).
- Temazepam, although it can lead to neonatal withdrawal, is safe when used alone. However, it has caused in utero death when taken with diphenhydramine, which is present in several over-the-counter preparations (e.g. Nytol, Benylin).

Drugs for Skin Diseases

- Topical creams are safe.
- First trimester use of prednisolone and other systemic steroids might increase the risk of cleft lip and cleft palate, so use topical steroids or keep systemic courses short. Topical steroids carry the same kind of risks as systemic steroids but are safer because you just don't absorb that much. For example, a pregnant woman getting through one 30 g tube of Betnovate a week would only be exposing her fetus to the equivalent of 17 mg hydrocortisone a day, which, although being a 'physiological dose', is unlikely to cause problems.
- Isotretinoin capsules cause defects in about one-third of all babies exposed in the first trimester. There is a recognised pattern of defects involving cardiac and craniofacial abnormalities. Acitretin, another vitamin A analogue, carries the same risk as excess vitamin A in pregnancy.

The Basic Principles of Prescribing and Breastfeeding

Alia Husain

Prescribing in breastfeeding is quite a specialist field, where the evidence base is far from exhaustive. Check with your registrar/consultant and pharmacist! Make sure that you know about the medicines you are prescribing and understand the need.

The Basic Rules

Keep it SIMPLE. Don't ever prescribe unless absolutely necessary. Most mums will happily put up with a headache rather than take paracetamol. However, there are some cases where drugs must be given but breastfeeding is contraindicated, e.g. in those taking anticancer agents.

Select the CLASS of drug that you want to use. Now select the drug with the shortest half-life, the most evidence-based information with the smallest number of side effects.

Look for those drugs that require a *once-daily* administration. This gives the mother the option to feed or express when levels of the drug are at their lowest.

Ask yourself:

- How much drug is getting into the milk?
- What are the associated risks to the infant?

The BNF is insufficient, so also ask your pharmacist/medicines information team.

Inform the parents of side effects to look out for. While the majority of antibiotics are safe in breastfeeding, they *will* cross into the milk and may cause the baby to have loose or increased stools.

If a treatment decreases the amount of breast milk being produced (e.g. diuretics), recommend more visits to the breast rather than topping up with infant formula. Explain to the mother that this needs to be balanced against an increased risk of nipple soreness.

If the mother must stop breastfeeding during a short course of treatment, suggest temporary options to her such as express and discard.

With acknowledgement to Fiona Maguire, who was the original author of this chapter.

Understanding the Reputable Literature

Drugs are often classified in the following manner:

'Compatible with breastfeeding.'

Enough said.

'Compatible with breastfeeding. Monitor infant for side effects.'

Can theoretically cause side effects. They have either not been seen before or are minor in nature. Reassure, explain what to look out for and ask the mother to return if necessary.

'Avoid if possible. Monitor infant for side effects.'

Often the drug has been reported to cause a serious side effect. Only use if absolutely necessary and where there is nothing else available. Arrange regular follow-ups to support monitoring. A decision might need to be taken to stop therapy.

'Avoid if possible. May inhibit lactation.'

Try to avoid, especially if it will have a negative impact upon the mother's psychological well-being. This effect can be countered by regular trips to the breast.

'Avoid.'

If this is the only option for treatment, seek specialist help. The issues of not breastfeeding need to be explained, and other people will have more experience than you.

'Safe' Drugs

Drugs that are safe to give in normal adult doses to the mother of a normal term infant include:

- *Antibiotics*: penicillins, cephalosporins, erythromycin (there is more evidence with this than clarithromycin) and gentamicin, provided you have understood the section on Therapeutic Drug Monitoring (see Chapter 37).
- *NSAIDs*: first line – ibuprofen, second line – naproxen are the drugs of choice.
- *Asthma therapy*: all inhalers, theophylline.
- *Non-sedating antihistamines*: e.g. cetirizine.
- *Corticosteroids*: lower doses of short courses of prednisolone e.g. ≤30 mg daily.
- *Beta-blockers*: labetalol is the drug of choice. Most of the others will pass to the milk and cause all sorts of side effects in the baby, including bradycardia and hypotension.

- *Laxatives*: senna, lactulose and Fybogel are suitable as they are not absorbed from the GI tract. Avoid co-danthramer.
- *Low molecular weight heparins*: dalteparin and enoxaparin are safe.

Caution Required

Drugs to be used with caution (i.e. use minimum dose possible) include:

- *Opioid analgesics and antipsychotics*: use these in the lowest possible doses and warn the mother to look out for sedation and to stop breastfeeding if the baby becomes very sleepy. Avoid high doses and avoid lithium. There is an MHRA alert to avoid codeine completely in breastfeeding mothers due to a case of morphine toxicity in a breastfed baby.
- *Anticonvulsants*: sodium valproate and carbamazepine. Apart from these, other anticonvulsants might need to be used in exceptional circumstances because of the needs of the mother. The baby will need to be monitored and there is little published data.
- *Antidepressants*: e.g. non-sedating tricyclics and SSRIs are used in postnatal depression. Risk/benefit analysis usually favours prescribing, but watch out for growth problems and irritability. May cause developmental problems.

Avoid if Possible

Avoid breastfeeding if at all possible (discuss with consultant):

- drugs of abuse
- high-dose sedative drugs
- certain immunosuppressants.

Always Avoid

Drugs that should always lead the patient to avoid breastfeeding:

- cytotoxic agents
- radioactive substances.

Management of the Delirious (Acutely Confused) Patient

Jim Bolton

What is Delirium?

Delirium is a state of global disturbance of cerebral function. It is characterised by altered conscious level (e.g. clouding of consciousness, drowsiness, attentional deficit), cognitive dysfunction (e.g. disorientation, memory impairment) and abnormalities in thinking (e.g. delusions), perception (e.g. illusions and hallucinations), mood and the sleep–wake cycle. It has an acute onset, hence it is often referred to as 'acute confusion' and it runs a fluctuating course. Behaviour in delirium can be hyperactive, hypoactive or both (mixed). It can be difficult to distinguish delirium from dementia and the two commonly co-exist.

Delirium is common in a general hospital, affecting over 30% of inpatients. Rates are particularly high in older adults, postoperative and intensive care patients, those with diseases of the central nervous system and in the context of terminal illness.

What Causes Delirium?

Delirium is caused by a sufficiently severe insult to the brain. It is the final common pathway of many causes, often in combination, including:

- Underlying medical conditions
- Drug treatments (e.g. anticholinergics, sedatives, opiates, steroids)
- Alcohol and substance misuse/withdrawal.

Commonly it is due to multiple seemingly minor causes in a vulnerable individual. Occasionally the cause is not identified, but the clinical picture is clearly that of delirium.

Vulnerability to delirium is generally greatest in children, who have an immature brain, and older adults, due to age-related diminished cerebral reserve. Vulnerability is greater still in those with dementia.

Assessment of the Delirious Patient

Key areas to enquire about include:

- The time course and pattern of confusion – delirium will typically have an acute onset and run a fluctuating course
- Past medical history – including identification of factors that might contribute to the current presentation; past history of confusion, acute or chronic
- Alcohol and/or substance misuse – could the presentation be contributed to by intoxication or a withdrawal state?
- A review of the patient's drug chart to identify any drugs that have been recently prescribed or withdrawn, or where the dose has been altered, and which might be contributing to delirium.

History from a delirious patient may be absent or unreliable, hence collateral information is often important in establishing the diagnosis from sources such as medical records, family, carers and the patient's GP.

Initial Management of the Delirious Patient

Priorities include:

- Treating the underlying causes
- Minimising polypharmacy and use of drugs that might contribute to the patient's confusion
- Providing a suitable care environment, e.g. a side room that minimises over-stimulation, and providing familiar staffing
- Ensuring effective communication and reorientation, e.g. minimising sensory impairment by ensuring that the patient has their glasses and a functioning hearing aid, and providing them with a clock and calendar
- Reassuring family and carers and explaining to them what is happening. They often play a valuable role in reorientating and calming an anxious patient.

Drug Treatment for Delirium

Drug treatments for delirium, usually considered to help calm an agitated patient, should be avoided if possible, as they have significant potential adverse effects. They should be used after consideration of the balance of risks, when de-escalation techniques are insufficiently effective and when the patient is judged to pose a significant risk to themselves or others or is very distressed.

The exception to this is when the delirium is caused by or contributed to by acute alcohol withdrawal (delirium tremens) in which case a benzodiazepine detoxification regimen should be initiated to minimise the risk of potentially dangerous complications, e.g. withdrawal seizures (see Chapter 8 – Prevention of Delirium Tremens and Management of Alcohol Withdrawal Syndrome).

The choice of drug treatment for other patients with delirium is usually between a benzodiazepine and an antipsychotic. The National Institute for Health and Care Excellence (2010) found little evidence for the use of drug treatments in delirium, but the best available evidence was for haloperidol. The most commonly used drugs worldwide are probably lorazepam and haloperidol.

General Advice on Prescribing

- Consider whether PRN rather than regular medication is sufficient.
- Give oral medication if possible before prescribing parenteral treatment.
- Start at the lowest clinically appropriate dose of a drug.
- Titrate cautiously according to symptoms.
- Regularly review the need for medication, the dose required, and the presence of adverse effects.
- Use for the shortest possible time, ideally one week or less.

Antipsychotics

- Antipsychotic drugs should be used with caution or not at all in patients with Parkinson's disease or Lewy body dementia, because of the high risk of exacerbating extrapyramidal symptoms.
- Antipsychotics carry an increased risk of cerebral ischaemia, stroke and increased mortality when prescribed for people with dementia, but the significance of this with short-term use is uncertain.
- Haloperidol has the potential to increase the QTc interval and precipitate life-threatening arrhythmia. An ECG to confirm a normal QTc should be taken before haloperidol is prescribed. If this is impractical, then consider use of a benzodiazepine instead. If haloperidol is prescribed without a screening ECG, this should be performed once the patient is sufficiently settled.

Benzodiazepines

- A benzodiazepine, such as lorazepam, may be effective for lesser degrees of agitation.
- Short-term use of a hypnotic may be appropriate for a patient whose main problem is disturbed nights.
- Potential adverse effects include excessive sedation, a worsening of confusion, unsteadiness and falls.

Prognosis

Delirium may take several weeks to resolve, long after the underlying causes have been treated and investigations have returned to normal, especially in patients with pre-existing cognitive impairment. For some patients, an episode of delirium may be followed by an irreversible degree of cognitive impairment. The mortality of delirious patients is twice that of non-delirious patients with similar medical conditions. Delirium is also associated with persistent functional decline, poorer rehabilitation, institutionalisation and rehospitalisation. Hence, delirium should be screened for, prevented where possible and treated when it occurs.

Further Reading

- National Institute for Health and Care Excellence. Delirium: Prevention, Diagnosis and Management (CG103), 2010. www.nice.org.uk/guidance/cg103 (accessed January 2020).

- A patient information leaflet on delirium is available on the Royal College of Psychiatrists website: www.rcpsych.ac.uk/expertadvice/problemsdisorders/delirium.aspx (accessed January 2020).

Chapter

8

Prevention of Delirium Tremens and Management of Alcohol Withdrawal Syndrome

Robert Shulman

Do not take alcohol withdrawal lightly. It can be lethal through its physiological consequences, direct injury (such as jumping from a window) or non-compliance (such as pulling out chest drains or drips). Find out what local facilities are available for longer-term management of alcohol dependence. The following guidelines are for inpatients only.

In dealing with alcohol dependence and withdrawal, there are two headlines:

Headline 1: Think of Drink!
- Always, ALWAYS, ALWAYS ask about alcohol consumption – and make it clear that you are non-judgemental. Remember to be suspicious: assume that most people (just like you!) underestimate their consumption.
- Look for clues that there might be an alcohol problem. Is the MCV high? Are there healed fractures on chest X-ray? Is there a history compatible with excess intake?

Headline 2: A Preventative Measure
A heavy drinker, deprived of alcohol for a day or two, *will* get the DTs. Guaranteed. This usually happens between days 2 and 5, but can come on earlier (e.g. ≤24 hours). You have four choices when dealing with the dependent:

1. Discuss the issue, and allow them to drink responsibly while in hospital, if this fits with the pattern of investigation, local practices and treatment.

2. Prescribe a steady background of medication to stop them withdrawing from alcohol.

3. Prescribe a reducing dose of medication so that they safely withdraw from alcohol (if they'd like to stop drinking).

4. Watch like a hawk for worrying signs: rising pulse rate, tremor, sweatiness, agitation and ACT SMARTLY TO TREAT.

With acknowledgement to the UCLH guidelines.

Drug Management of Delirium Tremens

Remember that 'one size doesn't fit all'. Sedative doses should be tailored to the individual requirements. This requires review at least once daily.

Preventing and Managing DTs

There are a variety of regimens available for this purpose. However, chlordiazepoxide is the drug of choice, though in severe hepatic impairment or cirrhosis lorazepam could be used as it is shorter acting. Initially, chlordiazepoxide 30 mg QDS should be adequate, but in severe cases, increase the dose to a maximum of 50 mg QDS. For night time sedation, give a larger dose, e.g. double the daytime dose at bedtime and the ward will enjoy a quieter night! Take care when prescribing for a patient who is intoxicated or sedated.

If you opt for controlled withdrawal, Table 8.1 shows a suggested oral reducing regimen (titrate according to the patient's response).

Prescribe the same dose PRN on top of this.

Doses can be reduced if necessary, such as in elderly patients.

Benzodiazepines at Discharge

Generally, these should not be prescribed at discharge. However, if the patient is part of a detox programme and is low risk for alcohol consumption after discharge then consider a regimen on chlordiazepoxide such as: 10 mg QDS for one day, 5 mg QDS for one day, 5 mg BD for one day.

Table 8.1 Chlordiazepoxide reducing dose table

Severity	Admin time	Day 1	Day 2	Day 3	Day 4	Day 5
Mild	06⁰⁰	20 mg	10 mg	5 mg	5 mg	
	12⁰⁰	20 mg	10 mg	5 mg		
	18⁰⁰	20 mg	10 mg	5 mg		
	24⁰⁰	20 mg	10 mg	5 mg	5 mg	5 mg
Moderate	06⁰⁰	30 mg	20 mg	10 mg	5 mg	5 mg
	12⁰⁰	30 mg	20 mg	10 mg	5 mg	
	18⁰⁰	30 mg	20 mg	10 mg	5 mg	
	24⁰⁰	30 mg	20 mg	10 mg	5 mg	5 mg
Severe	06⁰⁰	40 mg	30 mg	20 mg	10 mg	5 mg
	12⁰⁰	40 mg	30 mg	20 mg	10 mg	
	18⁰⁰	40 mg	30 mg	20 mg	10 mg	
	24⁰⁰	40 mg	30 mg	20 mg	10 mg	5 mg

Alternatives to Chlordiazepoxide

- Lorazepam has a shorter duration of action than chlordiazepoxide and may be preferable in elderly patients or those with severe hepatic dysfunction (0.5 mg lorazepam ~ 15 mg chlordiazepoxide).
- Diazepam should be used if the parenteral or rectal routes are required (5 mg diazepam ~ 15 mg chlordiazepoxide).
- Whichever drug and regimen you use, think of a larger dose last thing at night, reduce doses if sleepy and increase if signs of DTs are escalating.

Adjuncts to Chlordiazepoxide

Continue any established antiepileptic drugs. For patients who are not on any anticonvulsants but who are known to be susceptible to seizures, prescribe carbamazepine 200 mg PO 12-hourly during detoxification. Use diazepam 10 mg IV/PR STAT if chlordiazepoxide does not adequately control seizures. Consider propranolol 40 mg PO OD up to TDS PRN for reducing sweating, palpitations and tremor if the patient is particularly distressed.

Treating Acute Severe DTs

See Chapter 7 – Management of the Delirious Patient.

Prevention of Wernicke–Korsakoff Syndrome

REMEMBER: This condition can cause permanent disability. Prevent it!
On admission, administer parenteral Pabrinex® (containing vitamins B and C) to all alcohol-dependent patients who are due to undergo inpatient alcohol withdrawal, or to those patients who are thought to be severely thiamine deficient. You are using Pabrinex for the thiamine content. Pabrinex should be administered before any parenteral glucose is given.

Prevention of Wernicke's encephalopathy:

ONE pair of Pabrinex® IV high potency (HP) ampoules OD for 3–5 days.

Therapeutic treatment for Wernicke's encephalopathy:

TWO pairs of Pabrinex® IVHP ampoules TDS for 3 days, then OD for 5 days. If no response is seen, discontinue therapy; if a response is seen, decrease the dose to ONE pair of ampoules daily, given for as long as improvement continues.

When the Pabrinex course is finished, give oral thiamine 100 mg BD and 1 multivitamin tablet daily, usually for the rest of the admission and on discharge.

Chapter

Diabetic Ketoacidosis
Lloyd E. Kwanten

9

Diabetic ketoacidosis (DKA) is a life-threatening state of absolute or relative insulin deficiency aggravated by ensuing hyperglycemia, dehydration and deranged metabolism, producing ketoacidosis. The most common causes are underlying infection, disruption of insulin treatment and new onset of diabetes. Though it is more common in Type 1 diabetes, it can also occur in Type 2 diabetes.

For DKA to be diagnosed, the following criteria must be fulfilled:

- Known history of diabetes OR capillary blood glucose >11 mmol/L
- pH <7.3 or bicarbonate <15 on blood gas measurement (venous or arterial)
- Ketonaemia ≥3 mmol/L OR 2+ on urine dipstick.

Fluid replacement and intravenous insulin administration are the primary and most critical initial treatments of DKA. Subcutaneous insulin and oral fluids may be given in mild cases of DKA (where the patient is alert, not vomiting and not clinically dehydrated). More severe cases (especially in children) may need to be cared for in high-dependency units, and an early referral to specialist paediatrics, endocrinology or diabetes services is important. Emergency departments should make use of clinical pathways to reduce potential harmful errors in the management of DKA (e.g. the Joint British Diabetes Societies (JBDS) for Inpatient Care Guidelines available at https://abcd.care).

TOP TIPS for Prescribing in Adults with Severe DKA

- *Fluids*: Judicious fluid therapy is important as these patients are invariably volume deplete. Excess fluid administration may cause cerebral oedema; fluid use should be meticulously prescribed in paediatric, elderly, pregnant or cardiac and renal failure patients. In adults, give an initial fluid bolus of 1 L NaCl 0.9%, with subsequent fluids (e.g. NaCl 0.9% or Plasmalyte148) and rate based on clinical state, serum sodium and patient weight.   *(cont.)*

With acknowledgement to Preet Panesar, who was the original author of this chapter.

- *Insulin*: Soluble insulin (e.g. human Actrapid®) diluted to a concentration of 1 IU/mL administered with a syringe driver. STAT dose of 0.1 IU/kg IV, then infuse with a fixed-rate insulin infusion (FRII) at 0.1 IU/kg/hour. NICE guidelines do not recommend giving an IV bolus dose in paediatric populations. If the patient is already on a long-acting insulin, this should not be stopped. Blood glucose levels should be checked at least hourly, with the aim to reduce blood glucose by 2–4 mmol/L/hour. Once recovered from ketosis or acidosis, the patient can transition from an FRII to a variable-rate insulin infusion (VRII) insulin (see Chapter 35 – Intravenous Insulin Infusions). When able to eat and drink, subcutaneous insulin can be used, and the VRII should be discontinued 30–60 minutes after this is given.

- *Glucose*: In DKA, the hyperglycaemia is corrected faster than the ketoacidosis, so when blood glucose falls to less than 14 mmol/L, intravenous glucose 5% or 10% should be used in addition to the NaCl 0.9% infusion, as guided by fluid status.

- *Potassium*: Avoid potassium replacement with the first 1–2 L of fluid, if the potassium level >5.5 mmol/L or the patient is anuric. Check the serum K$^+$ every 2 hours for the first 6 hours, reducing in frequency after this. If K$^+$ <3.5 mmol/L, senior advice is required. The total potassium replacement in adults is likely to be 200–300 mmol over 24–48 hours.

TOP TIPS to Avoid Ketoacidosis

After an episode of DKA, counselling with the patient (and their family or carers) will prevent future episodes of DKA and readmission:

- Advise patients that good blood glucose control is the best way to keep blood glucose levels low enough to avoid DKA.

- If a patient becomes unwell, even if they are not eating, they should continue their insulin at the normal dose.

- Patients should be advised to test their blood at least four times a day or even more frequently if unwell. The urine may be tested for the presence of ketones.

- Advise your patients about the symptoms of hyperglycaemia and ketoacidosis, and if the capillary glucose results are high, they might need to increase their insulin dose, or check with their local diabetic team.

- If the patient cannot eat solid foods, tell them to replace them with alternatives, such as electrolyte or sugary drinks, or oral glucose tablets.

Hyperosmolar Hyperglycaemic State

Lloyd E. Kwanten

Hyperosmolar hyperglycaemic state (HHS), previously known as hyperosmolar non-ketotic coma (HONC), is usually seen in uncontrolled Type 2 diabetes. These patients tend to have severe dehydration, developing over many days, with a high blood glucose level (often over 40 mmol/L) without significant hyperketonaemia or acidosis. The majority of cases occur in middle-aged or elderly patients, usually with a concomitant illness, and two-thirds of cases occur in previously undiagnosed diabetics. It is a life-threatening emergency, and although less common than diabetic ketoacidosis (DKA), the mortality rate can be 10 times higher. These patients usually need admission to an intensive care or high dependency area. Management principles are similar to those of DKA, but there are some subtle differences with treatment.

TOP TIPS for Prescribing in Adults with HHS

- *Fluids*: Immediate aims are to expand circulating volume and restore peripheral perfusion. Boluses of NaCl 0.9% IV should be used initially, with the aim of treatment to replace 50% of estimated fluid loss within the first 12 hours and the remainder in the following 12 hours. Initially, hourly monitoring of fluid status, serum electrolytes, glucose and osmolality ($2Na^+$ + glucose + urea) is essential. The aim is to achieve a gradual decline in osmolality (3–8 mosmol/kg/hour) and normalisation may take up to 72 hours. Once blood glucose falls below 14 mmol/L, intravenous glucose 5% or 10% at 125 mL/hour should be commenced, in addition to the NaCl 0.9% infusion. Consider switching to NaCl 0.45% solution if the osmolality is not declining despite adequate positive fluid balance.

- *Insulin*: Insulin is not required initially. It should be commenced if there is co-existent ketonaemia or when serum glucose fails to fall with continued fluid replacement. Starting regimen is 0.05 IU/kg/hour with the aim to keep blood glucose at 10–15 mmol/L in first 24 hours.

(cont.)

With acknowledgement to Preet Panesar, who was the original author of this chapter.

- *Potassium*: Potassium requirements are much less than with DKA, and replacement should be guided by renal function and serum potassium levels.
- *Anticoagulation*: These patients are at an increased risk of venous thromboembolism and prophylactic low molecular weight heparin should be commenced.

Chapter 11

Hypoglycaemia

Lloyd E. Kwanten

Hypoglycaemia is defined as a blood glucose less than 4 mmol/L, although symptoms may only occur when blood glucose is much lower. Symptoms such as drowsiness, altered personality, poor concentration, sweating and confusion may go unnoticed by the patient and staff looking after them. Left untreated, hypoglycaemia can cause accidents, fits, permanent brain injury or even death. A variety of risk factors make hypoglycaemic episodes more likely in hospitals: irregular eating habits, delaying meals, 'nil by mouth', inability to absorb food, recent changes in medication and doses, and insulin dosing errors.

Episodes can be divided into mild to moderate or severe, and treatment depends on which category the patient falls into. Hypoglycaemia which causes unconsciousness is a medical emergency.

Conscious Patients with Mild to Moderate Hypoglycaemia (2.2–4 mmol/L)

- 15–20 g of glucose given orally (e.g. 5–7 Dextrosol® tablets, 4–5 Glucotabs®, 60 mL Glucojuice®, 150–200 mL pure fruit juice or 3–4 heaped teaspoons of sugar dissolved in water). Proprietary 40% glucose gels (Glucogel) can be squeezed inside the cheek and gently rubbed to allow absorption through the lining of the mouth.

- If blood glucose remains below 4 mmol/L after 15 minutes – repeat dose of oral glucose. If hypoglycaemia persists, IV glucose may need to be used (see next section).

- Once blood glucose is above 4 mmol/L, a long-acting (low glycaemic index) carbohydrate such as a sandwich, fruit or biscuits, will prevent recurrence of hypoglycaemia.

With acknowledgement to Preet Panesar, who was the original author of this chapter.

Unconscious Patients with Severe Hypoglycaemia (<2.2 mmol/L)

- Administer basic life support and seek urgent medical help.

- Glucagon 1 mg can be used, given by IV, IM or SC routes, which is an advantage if the patient is fitting or has no intravenous access. However, it is slower to act than IV glucose (it can take 10 minutes to see clinical improvement) and is ineffective in patients with low glycogen stores (e.g. starved patients, alcoholics, elderly and those with frequent hypoglycaemic episodes) and is not suitable for type 2 diabetics.

- Glucose IV: 100–200 mL of 10% glucose (or 50–100 mL of 20% glucose) should be infused through a wide-bore cannula (high-concentration glucose is an irritant to veins). Patients usually respond quickly and will need regular blood glucose monitoring.

- Once the blood glucose is greater than 4 mmol/L and the patient has recovered consciousness, a long-acting carbohydrate meal should be given (see previous section). Where the episode of hypoglycaemia is caused by insulin or a hypoglycaemic agent, the effects of these drugs may persist for many hours, and regular checking of blood glucose levels is required.

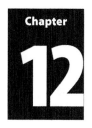
Chapter

12

Paracetamol Overdose
Mayur Murali

Paracetamol overdose is defined as ingestion of more than 4 g paracetamol in 24 hours. It is common and can prove fatal in adults: 10–15 g (20–30 tablets) can cause severe hepatocellular failure, acute renal tubular necrosis (more rarely) and then death 3 to 4 days later. It would be out of place to discuss management extensively here, but a few useful tips are given below.

There are two treatment strategies:

- Decreasing absorption
- Supporting non-toxic metabolism of the drug.

Decreasing Absorption

- Single dose of activated charcoal (50 g STAT) reduces paracetamol absorption ONLY if given within 2 hours of overdose.
- Routinely give antiemetics alongside.
- Reduce dose and raise frequency if still not tolerated (e.g. 25 g 2-hourly or 12.5 g hourly).

Metabolic Manipulation

N-Acetylcysteine (NAC) aids the metabolism of paracetamol down a non-hepatotoxin-producing pathway. Prescribe as an IV infusion in a 5% glucose solution:

- Initially 150 mg/kg in 200 mL 5% glucose over 1 hour THEN
- 50 mg/kg in 500 mL over 4 hours THEN
- 1000 mg/kg in 1000 mL over 16 hours.

With acknowledgement to Jane Ng, who was the original author of this chapter. **49**

If You Know When the Overdose Was Taken

Within 8 Hours of Overdose

- Take blood for paracetamol levels >4 hours following overdose (samples taken earlier are inaccurate).
- Refer to nomogram in BNF.
- Treat if above treatment 'normal' line, or if above 'high-risk' line if the patient is in a 'high-risk' category, i.e. in patients on enzyme-inducing drugs/malnourished (alcoholism, HIV), toxicity can develop at lower paracetamol levels.
- NAC may also be considered if biochemical tests suggest acute liver injury (e.g. ALT above upper limit of normal).
- Consider prescribing an antiemetic in vomiting patients.

Late Presentation (>8 Hours after Overdose)

- Treat with NAC at once
- Take level
- Continue treatment based on level and risk status.

Late (>24 Hours)

- As for >8 hours after overdose
- Take advice from liver unit.

If the Overdose was Staggered or of Unknown Timing

- Treat if in doubt. Give activated charcoal and NAC, and continue for >24 hours.
- Take blood for a paracetamol level at least 4 hours after the last paracetamol ingestion.
- Hepatotoxicity is unlikely if all the following apply: patient asymptomatic; serum paracetamol concentration <10 mg/L; INR <1.3; ALT in normal range.

When to Refer to a Liver Unit

Discuss EARLY with your liver unit, *before* metabolic acidosis, coagulopathy or encephalopathy occur. In general, transfer to a liver unit is indicated if:

- arterial lactate >3.5 mmol/L after fluid resuscitation
- arterial pH <7.3 AND lactate >3 mmol/L after fluid resuscitation
- PT/INR > 100s/6s AND encephalopathy grade ≥3 AND creatinine >292 μmol/L within 24 hours AND normal arterial pH.

TOP TIPS

- BEWARE the well patient who has taken a paracetamol overdose. Do NOT discharge. Admit, monitor and treat!
- Never take the word of a patient who has taken an overdose: they may well have taken a far greater dose than they recollect.
- Always screen for other drugs that they might have taken too – especially salicylates.
- Do NOT correct an abnormal INR without having talked with the liver unit – it can be the best guide to decline and need for transplant.
- In pregnancy, use the patient's prepregnancy weight for the toxic dose and the actual weight for the NAC dose.
- For patients weighing more than 110 kg, the toxic dose and the NAC dose should be calculated using a maximum of 110 kg rather than the patient's actual weight.

Emergency Prescribing in Cardiology

Sebastian Vandermolen
and David Brull

Acute Coronary Syndromes

Acute coronary syndromes (ACS) represent partial or complete clot occlusion of a coronary artery. They present as anginal chest pain at rest or on mild exertion, with or without either ECG changes or rise in cardiac enzymes.

All generally receive:

- *Analgesia with antiemetic:*
  - diamorphine 2.5–5 mg IV/SC PRN
  - metoclopromide 10 mg PO/IV/IM TDS

- *Antiplatelet agents:*
  - aspirin 300 mg PO STAT, then 75 mg PO OD
  - clopidogrel 300 mg PO STAT, then 75 mg PO OD

  OR

- Ticagrelor 180 mg PO loading dose STAT, followed by 90 mg BD

(Consider a PPI, especially in the elderly.)

> Ticagrelor has a more rapid onset of antiplatelet activity than clopidogrel. It is associated with lower rates of death, non-fatal MI or stroke after an initial ACS episode (PLATO trial), but with higher rates of intracranial and GI bleeding, and premature discontinuation.

- *Beta-blocker (blood pressure allowing): bisoprolol 2.5–10 mg PO OD once stable*
  - Beware asthma, acute LVF, low BP, low HR, 2nd/3rd degree heart block.
  - If contraindicated, if blood pressure allows, consider slow-release diltiazem if no signs of heart failure

- *Strict glycaemic control for diabetics if CBGs above 11 mmol/L*
  - In the first instance consider a dose-adjusted insulin infusion
- *IV fluids if RV infarct* – clues include low BP with no pulmonary oedema, raised JVP, posterior/inferior ST changes.

If STEMI

- Liaise with the nearest PCI centre and arrange emergency transfer.
- Urgently discuss patients who are unfit or unstable for immediate transfer (e.g. haemodynamic instability, stroke with dense hemiplegia, acute confusion, major co-morbidity).
- If transfer for PCI is unavailable, thrombolyse (unless contraindicated) within 30 minutes of diagnosis.

If NSTEMI

- 2.5 mg fondaparinux OD SC for 5 days.

Secondary Prevention

- Dual antiplatelets for one year
- Beta-blocker and ACE inhibitor
- Add mineralcorticoid receptor antagonist (MRA) in established LVF with EF <40%
- Check lipids, add statin
- Check HbA1c
- Diet/lifestyle/smoking cessation/cardiac rehab as appropriate.

Acute Severe Pulmonary Oedema

For all:

- *High-flow oxygen* (monitor oxygen saturations and arterial blood gases)
- *Opiate with antiemetic:*
  - diamorphine 2.5–5 mg IV/SC PRN
  - metoclopramide 10 mg PO/IV/IM TDS
- *Nitrate infusion titrating to BP* (50 mg in 50 mL of normal saline, initially 2 mL/hour but titrated to pain and systolic BP >90–100 mmHg)
- *Consider furosemide* (particularly if fluid overloaded: 40–80 mg IV STAT)

If patient doesn't respond:

- Discuss with ICU early!
- If cardiogenic shock is present, discuss with tertiary cardiology referral centre; this is now mandatory.

Further specific therapy will depend on the cause or exacerbating factors of failure. Consider:

- ACS, valvular heart disease, cardiomyopathy
- Infection, arrhythmia, uraemia

TOP TIPS for the Management of Acute Pulmonary Oedema

- Hold beta-blockers, unless failure is rate-related, e.g. fast AF, high rate in hypertrophic cardiomyopathy, mitral stenosis.
- CPAP or BIPAP can be additional therapeutic measures.
- Mechanical ventilation and inotropes (e.g. dobutamine) might be required.

Arrhythmias

For any of the tachyarrhythmias, if the patient is haemodynamically compromised, EMERGENCY DC CARDIOVERSION should be considered. Remember to 'synchronise' the defibrillator to avoid the 'R on T' phenomenon.

Supraventricular Tachycardia

Don't panic – SVTs are usually well tolerated! Set up continuous ECG monitoring. First-line therapies include:

- Vagal manoeuvres – carotid sinus massage, Valsalva (new research suggests best results when legs raised – known as modified Valsalva)
- Failing that, try adenosine:
  - Warn patient about chest tightness/flushing: this lasts <20 seconds.
  - Using a large vein, followed by a rapid bolus of saline flush, inject bolus adenosine 3 mg, 6 mg, 9 mg, then 12 mg, allowing 30 seconds between increments to assess for response.
  - Adenosine will terminate the tachycardia or cause transient AV block, which will help to diagnose the underlying atrial rhythm (usually flutter if doesn't cease completely).
- In asthmatics or if adenosine unsuccessful, consider verapamil 2.5–5 mg IV (do not use in patients receiving beta-blockers).

Adenosine

Contraindicated: asthma

Caution:

- heart transplant (reduce dose)
- AF (increases accessory pathway)
- prolonged QTc
- COPD (bronchospasm)

Warn: transient unpleasant feeling, facial flushing, dyspnoea

If the above fails to terminate the tachycardia or has only a transient effect, try an AV node blocker:

- *Digoxin*: load with 500 mg two doses PO 4-hourly, then 250 mg PO OD (doesn't need to be given IV); or
- *Flecainide*: 2 mg/kg IV over 30 minutes (monitor for AV block); or
- *Sotalol*: 80 mg PO BD
- *Amiodarone* can be used, but has a slow mode of onset orally and requires central IV infusion because of the risk of phlebitis.

Ventricular Tachycardia (Non-Pulseless)

Confirm the ECG diagnosis. If you are unclear whether this is VT or SVT, try vagal manoeuvres or adenosine, as above.

Treat correctable factors:

- Aim for $K^+ > 4.5$ mmol/L
- Then, infuse IV Mg^{2+} 8 mmol over 15 minutes, then 72 mmol over 24 hours.

Consider (the following can all cause hypotension and aggravate heart failure):

- *Beta-blockers*, e.g. metoprolol 25 mg PO TDS (short-acting, so quick wash-out if hypotension occurs)
- *Amiodarone* IV 300 mg over 30 minutes, then 900 mg over 24 hours via a large central vein

    OR

- Overdrive pacing

Remember, pulseless VT = VF = *IMMEDIATE DEFIBRILLATION*!

Emergency Prescribing in Neurosurgery

Sheetal Sumaria and
Lindsey Stockford

The neurosurgical patient is not normally one that you should be caring for in a non-specialist bed, but you may find yourself looking after such a patient while the referral is being made. The neurosurgical registrar will advise you with management. Remember to communicate to them *any changes* in the patient's neurological state, as a change in therapy might be required. You will only be asked to do a few things. Here are some top tips to help you.

Subarachnoid Haemorrhage

By and large, these will be caused by the rupture of an intracranial artery. As a result:

- If you are conscious, *it hurts!*
- Intracranial pressure (ICP) can rise from generalised cerebral oedema secondary to the insult, and/or compression of the ventricular system by a resultant cerebral haematoma. This can reduce cerebral blood flow and cause cerebral ischaemia.
- Blood swilling around in cerebrospinal fluid causes spasm of the large arteries in the base of the brain, resulting in even worse cerebral ischaemia.
- The vessel can rebleed.

Immediate management is thus geared towards pain relief, maintaining cerebral perfusion (reducing ICP and limiting vasospasm) and reducing the risk of rebleeding.

Blood Pressure Control

Reactive arterial hypertension is common, and helps maintain cerebral perfusion in the face of a raised ICP. But, too high a blood pressure and the risk of rebleeding increases, while too low a blood pressure will exacerbate cerebral ischaemia. Then there is the patient's usual blood pressure to consider: someone

---

normally hypertensive needs a higher blood pressure now than a past normotensive. So what blood pressure *do* you aim for? As always, ask your neurosurgeon to guide you. Meanwhile, some basic dos and don'ts are given in Table 14.1.

Table 14.1 Dos and don'ts of blood pressure control in subarachnoid haemorrhage

Do	Don't
Have the patient 'head up 30°'	Treat in order to get a 'normal BP', or be worried by even moderately raised MAP. As a rule of thumb, aim for 20% higher than baseline BP (if known)
Treat the pain! Start with paracetamol 1 g PO/NG/PR/IV QDS regularly. You can also use short-acting morphine sulfate (e.g. morphine sulfate 5 mg PO 3 hourly PRN) or small doses (1–2 mg repeated doses) SC if the patient is vomiting. Small doses don't compromise neuro-assessment	Use an NSAID. The antiplatelet effect increases the risk of rebleeding
Get HDU/ICU involved if you're at all concerned about the patient's consciousness or BP. Gross hypertension should be treated with agents that can be 'switched off' – i.e. avoid tablets. The intensivist will consider a short-acting IV antihypertensive such as labetolol, or GTN. You should not have to do this	Reduce the MAP too fast or too dramatically. In general, do not use sublingual nifedipine, as the response is fast, unpredictable, sustained and hard to reverse. Speak to the neurosurgeon

And Remember Fluids!

· All SAH patients need enough fluid to counteract vasospasm. Keep them well hydrated!

· Giving fluid to an underfilled patient can help bring BP down (oddly enough!)

· The minimum fluid input should, in general, be 3 L of crystalloid in 24 hours.

· Avoid glucose-containing solutions as these can worsen cerebral oedema.

· Caution in elderly or patients with heart failure.

· If the patient becomes hypotensive, fluid challenge them with crystalloid.

If, in spite of this, the patient remains hypotensive, inotropes might be indicated: get HDU/ICU involved at this point!

Spasm

Nimodipine is a (supposedly cerebroselective) calcium-channel antagonist. It saves lives after SAH by reducing spasm. Prescribe it as 60 mg PO/NG 4 hourly. BP may fall (as, in fact, it opens up *all* blood vessels). If profound hypotension occurs after each dose, prescribe 30 mg PO/NG 2 hourly instead.

Rebleeding

- Give all SAH patients regular stool softeners (such as lactulose). Straining is a good way to have another bleed!
- DON'T use NSAIDs for pain.
- DON'T use low molecular weight heparin as VTE prophylaxis. Use graded compression stockings instead.

Bleeding and the Brain

In any cerebral bleed, or where one is likely:

- Don't give warfarin or DOACs. If on warfarin, reverse it (see Chapter 28 – Warfarin Prescribing); seek haematology advice about DOAC reversal/follow local guidance (see Chapter 30 – Direct Oral Anticoagulants).
- Avoid heparin VTE prophylaxis: use graded compression stockings instead.
- Avoid NSAIDs.
- Consider ulcer prophylaxis, as stress ulceration is common.

Steroids and Neurosurgery

Steroids will reduce swelling around tumours, relieving cord compression and lowering ICP. They will also reduce neuronal swelling associated with cauda equina compression secondary to a prolapsed disc. This can be treated with dexamethasone (doses can vary; usual range is up to 16 mg daily in divided doses, and dose is usually reduced depending on indication and symptom control).

Steroid use in acute spinal injury is a contentious issue. Initial trials showed that methylprednisolone given within 8 hours of injury was beneficial. However, more recent data challenges this. Moreover, these trials suggest that steroid use might in fact be harmful. Ask the neurosurgeon what to do.

Mannitol and Neurosurgery

Mannitol is an osmotic diuretic. It can reduce ICP and, in certain cases, is a useful temporary holding measure until the patient can be delivered to a neurosurgical unit for a definitive operative procedure. Only give on the instruction of a neurosurgeon.

Mannitol Methods

- Mannitol 20% comes in 500 mL bottles, which contain 100 g of drug.
- Dose: 20% mannitol 0.25–1.0 g/kg IV infusion over 15–20 minutes.
- In practice: *100 mL of mannitol 20% IV over 20 minutes.*
- Only repeat if instructed: it can paradoxically increase ICP.
- It will cause an osmotic diuresis. Catheterise! Watch electrolytes! Beware dehydration!

Anticonvulsants and Neurosurgery

Remember to ask. A fit is a very good way of making a brain injury worse by increasing brain metabolism, causing hypoxia (with the fit) and raising ICP (with all the thrashing around). Phenytoin or levetiracetam are often used (see Chapter 26 – Fit for a Fit). Prophylactic antiepileptics are rarely indicated.

TOP TIPS for Analgesia

- *Codeine* works by being converted to morphine; 5–10% of people can't do this at all, and about 30% do it badly. *Codeine is weak and its effects unreliable.*

- *If giving an opioid,* the dose needed will vary, according to patient tolerance.

- *Don't use non-steroidals* in patients where you want clotting to work properly – like those with subarachnoids!

Chapter 15

Respiratory Emergencies
Xolani Dereck Gondongwe

These usually manifest as bronchoconstriction and/or hypoxaemia and/or hypercapnia. The three primary management goals are:

- Optimise oxygenation and prevent carbon dioxide retention
- Determine the need for airway management and/or ventilator support
- Establish causes and initiate treatment.

This guide will focus on strategies to optimise oxygenation. Nearly all breathless patients (bar those with passive pulmonary embolus) benefit from sitting upright (where possible). This optimises ventilatory capacity and will also optimise inhaled drug therapy. Therefore, try and sit your patient upright. Below are some tips on what drugs need to be prescribed and how to prescribe them.

Hypoxaemia
Oxygen therapy improves oxygenation but does not treat the underlying cause of hypoxaemia, which must be diagnosed and treated as a matter of urgency. Oxygen has no consistent effect on breathlessness in non-hypoxaemic patients.
   For all critically ill patients:

- Prescribe and give oxygen at 15 L/min via a non-rebreathe mask until reliable oximetry readings are obtained. Aim for a target saturation range of 94–98%.

For seriously ill patients:

- If not at risk of CO_2 retention, prescribe and give oxygen at 15 L/min via a non-rebreathe mask. Aim for a target saturation range of 94–98%.
- If known to retain CO_2 (check for an oxygen alert card, previous ABGs, raised bicarbonate) or have signs consistent with CO_2 retention (bounding pulse, decreased GCS), aim for arterial blood oxygen saturation (SaO_2) of 88–92% until a blood gas can be analysed.
- If high oxygen concentrations are needed, discuss with critical care team about use of high-flow nasal oxygen (HFNO or 'Optiflow'), or admission to ICU for non-invasive or invasive ventilation.

With acknowledgement to Jane Ng, who was the original author of this chapter.

- Beware of overoxygenation, which may be harmful in other circumstances, including after head injury, cardiac arrest and in coronary vascular disease through vasoconstriction, oxidative stress and ultimately, cell death.

Tip 1 Oxygen must be prescribed. If using electronic prescribing, then familiarise yourself with template prescriptions. If using paper drug charts, the prescription is usually preprinted, so make sure that you know where to find this on the drug chart.

Tip 2 Revise the latest British Thoracic Guideline for oxygen use in adults in healthcare and emergency settings.

Bronchoconstriction
Inhaled Bronchodilators

Salbutamol (β_2 agonist) is the first-line inhaled bronchodilator, then ipratropium bromide (anticholinergic); combined, these drugs produce greater bronchodilation than a β_2 agonist alone (see Table 15.1).

Table 15.1 Inhaled bronchodilators

	Salbutamol	Ipratropium bromide
Dose	5 mg	500 micrograms
Frequency	Given STAT, then: If the patient is not improving, again after 15–30 minutes If the patient is improving, 4 hourly, with a PRN dose given every 2 hours	Given if life-threatening features are present Then, if the patient is not improving, 6 hourly until the patient improves
Mode	Nebuliser	Nebuliser

TOP TIPS for Nebulisation

- Ensure that the patient is sitting up, thereby increasing airway patency.
- The driving gas can either be oxygen or air (flow rate 6 L/min). In those with chronic obstructive pulmonary disease who are known or suspected to be oxygen sensitive (i.e. reliant on hypoxic ventilatory drive), use air-driven nebulisers. If the patient is at risk of desaturating without supplemental oxygen, then up to 6 L/min of oxygen can be supplied via nasal cannula with concomitant air-driven nebulised bronchodilators via face mask.
- In the absence of CO_2 retention, always use oxygen to drive the nebuliser for patients requiring supplemental oxygen.
- Always ensure that the driving gas for nebulised medication is specified on the prescription.

- Ask the patient to breathe through their mouth, preventing nasal deposition of the drug.
- Ask the patient if they would prefer a mouthpiece or face mask: ipratropium bromide is preferably given via a mouth piece, preventing ocular deposition and risk of glaucoma.
- Salbutamol and ipratropium bromide can be mixed and nebulised together.
- If the patient isn't tolerating nebulisers, try a spacer device: 1 puff of salbutamol from a metered dose inhaler = 100 micrograms (i.e. 5 mg dose = 50 puffs). Perhaps give 10 puffs into the spacer, asking the patient to take 10 deep breaths, then repeat four more times. This is a good trick for kids, who may not like nebulisers.

Steroid Therapy

Steroids reduce mortality, relapses, subsequent hospital admission and requirement for β_2 agonist therapy in acute asthma, and can improve lung function, oxygenation and shorten recovery time in exacerbations of COPD. The earlier they are given the better. Steroid tablets are as effective as injected steroids, provided the patient can swallow and retain them.

- In exacerbations of asthma, *prescribe prednisolone 40–50 mg daily or IV hydrocortisone 100 mg every 6 hours.* Continue prednisolone for at least 5 days or until recovery.

- In exacerbations of COPD, *prescribe 30 mg prednisolone daily.*

    Tip 3 Do not stop inhaled corticosteroids during prescription of oral corticosteroids. Doses do not need tapering provided the patient receives inhaled corticosteroids (apart from patients on maintenance steroid therapy or rare instances where steroids are required for 3 or more weeks).

Intravenous Bronchodilators

Magnesium Sulfate

There is some evidence that magnesium sulfate has bronchodilator effects. Therefore, consider giving a single dose of IV magnesium to patients with acute severe asthma (PEFR <50% best or predicted) who have not had a good initial response to inhaled bronchodilator therapy.

- *Prescribe magnesium sulfate 1.2–2 g IV infusion over 20 minutes.*

    Tip 4 Should only be used following consultation with senior medical staff.

Aminophylline

Aminophylline is the intravenous form of theophylline and is available in 250 mg (10 mL) ampoules. The latest British Thoracic Society guidelines (2019)[1] state that the addition of IV aminophylline in acute asthma is unlikely to result in additional bronchodilation not already achieved with standard therapy. It also has a raft of side effects, causing arrhythmias and vomiting. Though it may have benefit in patients with near fatal or life-threatening asthma with poor response to initial therapy, such patients are rare and were not identified in a meta-analysis of trials. In addition, levels need to be taken prior to administration in those on theophylline. In summary, it should only ever be used after consultation with senior medical staff.

- *Loading dose (theophylline naïve patients) – give 5 mg/kg over 30 minutes, then infusion of 0.5–0.7 mg/kg/h*
- In obese patients, doses should be based on ideal body weight
- ECG monitoring required.

See the Therapeutic Drug Monitoring section (Chapter 37) for maintenance dosing and monitoring details.

Tip 5 Use IV aminophylline only after consultation with senior medical staff.

Salbutamol

IV salbutamol is indicated if life-threatening features of asthma are present or if patients have not responded to initial therapy.

- *Prescribe salbutamol 250 mg IV over 20 minutes.* Infusions can run at 1–20 mg/min according to response.

Half-life is short, so increased infusion causes a rapid response and toxic effects die away quickly when rates are reduced. Being a selective receptor agonist, general side-effects (tremor/agitation) are also far fewer!

Tip 6 Review the latest BTS guidelines on the management of asthma and NICE COPD guidelines.

---

[1] British Thoracic Society. SIGN 158. British guideline on the management of asthma. A national clinical guideline. 2019. www.brit-thoracic.org.uk/quality-improvement/guidelines/asthma/. Accessed August 2019.

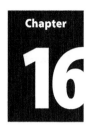

Pulmonary Embolism

Robert Shulman

Use the 'Wells score' (www.mdcalc.com/wells-criteria-pulmonary-embolism) to assess likelihood of PE and 'sPESI' (www.mdcalc.com/simplified-pesi-pulmonary-embolism-severity-index) to assess mortality risk.

Low-Risk PE

Anticoagulate with a low molecular weight heparin (LMWH), dependent on contraindications and bleeding risk. There are several LMWHs in use – find out the one used in your institution.

Remember to reduce the dose in renal impairment.

The patient may be suitable for discharge, and an oral agent (warfarin or DOAC) can be started in clinic. The INR target for warfarin is 2–3 and treatment should be continued for at least 3 months. See Chapter 28 – Warfarin Prescribing, and Chapter 30 – Direct Oral Anticoagulants.

Intermediate-Risk PE

This is an acute PE with normal blood pressure but evidence of myocardial necrosis or right ventricular dysfunction.

Initial treatment is with treatment dose LMWH, as per 'low-risk PE' above. Thrombolysis is considered if there is haemodynamic decompensation. In this case, treat as per 'high-risk PE' below.

High-Risk PE

High risk is defined here as an acute PE with sustained hypotension (SBP ≤ 90 mmHg for at least 15 min or requiring inotropic support, not due to a cause other than PE, such as arrhythmia, hypovolaemia, sepsis, or LV dysfunction), pulselessness or persistent profound bradycardia (pulse <40 bpm), with signs or symptoms of shock.

With acknowledgement to the UCLH guidelines.

Thrombolysis should be considered for high-risk PE. This and intermediate-risk PE will require a consultant review. Thrombolysis should be initiated without delay if there are no contraindications.

Thrombolysis

- *Alteplase*: IV 1.5 mg/kg (10 mg IV bolus stat, with remaining dose over 2 h, max. dose 100 mg).

  OR

- *Alteplase*: 50 mg IV bolus (patients with confirmed or imminent cardiac arrest).

If alteplase is still running, discontinue if a major bleed is suspected.

Anticoagulation Post Thrombolysis

Unfractionated heparin is increasingly no longer used in this scenario. LMWHs have largely superseded its use. Two hours after the end of thrombolysis, check APTT. If APTT <2 and CrCl ≥30 mL/min, start standard treatment PE dose, e.g. dalteparin 100 units/kg 12 hourly or enoxaparin 0.75 mg/kg BD. If APTT ≥2, repeat APTT every 4 hours until <2, then as above.

If anticoagulants were taken before thrombolysis, then delay the start of LMWH until the next dose is due, e.g. 12 hours after BD LMWH, 24 hours after treatment dose OD LMWH, at least 12 hours after BD apixaban (if CrCl ≥50 mL/min), at least 24 hours after rivaroxaban (if CrCl ≥50 mL/min).

Start warfarin on day 3–7 of LMWH therapy and continue until the INR is in the desired range for 2 consecutive days, with at least 5 days overlap.

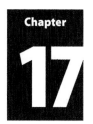

Chapter 17

Electrolyte and Metabolic Emergencies

Ned Gilbert-Kawai

A slow and steady increase or decrease in some electrolyte or other may go overlooked (or even consciously ignored) and can remain asymptomatic ('Who would have known?'). However, they can cause trouble insidiously ('Doc, I have a funny tingling around my mouth and lips'), or catastrophically (perhaps when causing an arrhythmia, or even cardiac arrest). So as a sagacious consultant once told me, 'don't delay and treat away'!

The Causes: Us and Them

THEM: Many conditions can lead to a poor intake of fluid and salts, loss of water and salts in varying quantities (e.g. stoma losses, diarrhoea, vomiting, sweat), or can directly affect handling of electrolytes (e.g. parathyroid disorders, renal disease, liver disease/heart failure, which activate the renin–angiotensin–aldosterone axis, adrenal dysfunction, vitamin D deficiency). Many of these can also affect acid–base balance directly (loss of acid in vomit, loss of bicarbonate in stool, problems with H^+ loss or bicarbonate resorption in renal diseases, liver failure meaning that lactate isn't broken down, or poor perfusion causing too much lactate to be made) or indirectly (e.g. hypokalaemia can cause an alkalosis).

US: We prescribe intravenous fluids without remembering that they are complex cocktails of water and different electrolytes, which can easily upset our blood chemistry. So 1 litre of 0.9% ('Normal') saline contains as much salt as 26 bags of crisps. Not what you'd choose if thirsty. It also contains 154 mmol of chloride, when blood contains only 100 mmol/L or so.

In EVERY patient, then, assess the total amount of water in every compartment (intravascularly empty or full? Tissue oedema or tissue dry?) and biochemical measures of dehydration/renal dysfunction (urea, creatinine), the concentration of salts, the *total amount*

With acknowledgement to Jane Ng, who was the original author of this chapter. **67** of those salts (i.e. someone may be salt and water overloaded and have a low [Na⁺] – and the last thing they need is more sodium!) and their acid/base status (serum bicarbonate, or an arterial blood gas if needs be). Then ask yourself does this patient need water and/or electrolytes? How much? And how much of which intravenous solution, or of what oral electrolyte supplement?

WHATEVER: Make a conscious decision on how often you should check a patient's bloods. Hourly (e.g. severe hyperkalaemia), 2–4 hourly (e.g. correcting severe hyponatraemia), twice daily (e.g. high-output fistula) or even daily (e.g. nil by mouth and on IV infusion).

Managing Trouble: The Rule of Three What's

1. *What's* the problem?

   If you spot a problem, how urgently does it need your undivided attention? Do the numbers make you yawn (minor change over a long time period), or sweat (major change over a short time period)? A potassium rising from 4.9 to 5.5 mmol/L over 3 days might prompt you to repeat the bloods later that day, while one of 8.3 mmol/L should demand your immediate and undivided attention – and quite possibly your urgent call to someone more senior.

2. *What's* causing it?

   Look at and around the patient, look at their medical history, and look at their associated notes, prescription charts and fluid prescription and balance charts. Stroke that metaphorical beard of yours and identify any disease (or treatment) that may be causing the problem.

3. *What* are you going to do about it?

   Stop medications and fluids which might be the cause. Test if you need e.g. short synacthen test/random blood cortisol, etc. Seek senior advise if unsure. And start any treatment you need – at once, if the abnormality is life-threatening.

Specific Management when GETTING HIGH!

Hyperkalaemia

When to worry: K⁺ is rising fast, is already >6.0 mmol/L, or ECG changes present (e.g. peaked T-waves, prolonged PR interval, widened QRS); see Table 17.1.

Table 17.1 Management of hyperkalaemia

Prescribe	Why?
Drug: 10% calcium gluconate or calcium chloride **Vol:** 10 mL **Route:** IV **Other:** Give over 2 minutes NB – some advocate only to give if ECG changes associated with hyperkalaemia: however, if in doubt, give it out	**Cardioprotection** High K⁺ destabilises cell transmembrane potential. Cardiac cells are particularly susceptible, and thus cardiac arrest can ensue
Drug: Actrapid insulin **Vol:** 5 units added to 50 mL of 50% glucose **Route:** IV **Other:** Give over 15 minutes	**Lowers plasma K⁺** Insulin drives K⁺ back into cells (and drops serum K⁺ by ~1 mmol/L in 30 minutes) Concurrent glucose administration is required to prevent hypoglycaemia
Drug: Salbutamol **Vol:** 10 mg **Route:** Nebuliser **Other:** Give over 5 minutes	**Lowers plasma K⁺** Increases cellular K⁺ uptake (and drops serum K⁺ by ~0.5 –1 mmol/L in 15 minutes).
Drug: Calcium resonium **Vol:** 15 g **Route:** PO (or, rarely, rectally) **Other:** TDS NB – always prescribe with lactulose (at least 10 mL TDS) as it is *extremely* constipating	**Binds K⁺** Binding K⁺ and promoting its excretion is a more definitive treatment (compared to the above)

ADDITIONALLY:

- Repeat bloods at about 2 hours or earlier if worried (VBG/ABG and send formal lab bloods)
- If the plasma K⁺ comes back still >6.0 mmol/L, consult a senior/the renal team/ICU/outreach team, as renal replacement therapy might be indicated
- Other measures:
  - 100 mL of 8.4% sodium bicarbonate IV over 10–20 minutes given through a large vein, *or*
  - 500 mL of 1.26% sodium bicarbonate IV over 1 hour.

These raise blood pH and therefore increase cellular K⁺ uptake

Hypercalcaemia

When to worry: A plasma Ca^{2+} is rising fast, is already >3.5 mmol/L, or ECG changes present (e.g. flattened T-waves, short QT and ST segments); (see Table 17.2).

Table 17.2 Management of hypercalcaemia

Prescribe	Why?
Drug: 0.9% sodium chloride **Vol:** May need 4–6 L (or much more) in 24 hours **Route:** IV **Other:** Monitor for fluid overload if renal impairment or elderly	**Rehydrate** These patients are almost always dry!
Drug: Zoledronic acid **Vol:** 4 mg **Route:** IV **Other:** Give over 15 minutes *Or* **Drug:** Pamidronate **Vol:** If plasma Ca^{2+} < 3 mmol/L: 30 mg If Ca^{2+} 3–3.5 mmol/L: 60 mg If Ca^{2+} > 3.5 mmol/L: 90 mg **Route:** IV **Other:** Give at 20 mg/h NB – give more slowly and consider dose reduction in renal impairment	**Limits endogenous Ca^{2+} release from bone stores** Through inhibiting osteoclastic activity, this is the most effective way of lowering Ca^{2+}. Will reach nadir at 2–4 days, and last 2–4 weeks

ADDITIONALLY:

- Repeat bloods at about 4 hours (VBG/ABG and send formal lab bloods)
- If the plasma Ca^{2+} comes back still >3.5 mmol/L, consult a senior/the renal team/ICU/outreach team as renal replacement therapy might be indicated
- IV bisphosphonates can cause hypocalcaemia if vitamin D deficient or suppressed PTH

Thyrotoxic Crisis or Thyroid Storm (A Rare Form of Acute Hyperthyroidism)

When to worry: Diagnosis is primarily clinical, including fever, tachycardia, hypertension, and neurological and gastrointestinal abnormalities. This may, however, progress rapidly to congestive heart failure and shock. Blood tests may show elevated T4 and T3, with suppressed TSH levels. See Table 17.3.

Table 17.3 Management of thyrotoxic crisis

Prescribe	Why?
Drug: Methimazole (MMI, thiamazole) **Vol:** 20 mg **Route:** PO/NG **Other:** 6-hourly (can give 30 mg/day, IV) *Or* **Drug:** Propylthiouracil (PTU) **Vol:** 200 mg **Route:** PO/NG **Other:** 4-hourly	**Prevents further synthesis of thyroid hormone** PTU also inhibits peripheral conversion of T4 to T3
Drug: Sodium iodide **Vol:** 1–2 g **Route:** IV **Other:** over 3–5 minutes (can give as IV infusion over 8–24 hours) *Or* **Drug:** Lugol's solution **Vol:** 0.3 mL **Route:** PO/NG **Other:** TDS NB – do not start until 1 hour after antithyroid drugs	**Inhibits thyroid function** Blocks the function of the thyroid gland by flooding it with iodine, and thus inhibits further thyroid hormone release
Drug: Propranolol **Vol:** 1 mg **Route:** IV **Other:** over 1 minute (can give as 40 mg PO/NG QDS) NB – repeat if needed up to 10 times at 2-minute intervals	**Ameliorates hyperadrenergic effects of thyroid hormone on peripheral tissues** And blocks T4 to T3 conversion in high doses
Drug: Hydrocortisone **Vol:** 100 mg **Route:** IV **Other:** TDS	**Prevents further thyroid hormone secretion and peripheral conversion of T4 to T3** Also provides prophylaxis against relative adrenal insufficiency

ADDITIONALLY:

- Beta$_1$-selective blockers (esmolol (IV), bisoprolol (PO)) should be the first choice of treatment for tachycardia in thyroid storm

- When atrial fibrillation occurs, digoxin is used in patients without severe renal dysfunction (initial dose is 125 to 250 mcg, IV). Alternatives to digoxin include calcium-channel blockers such as diltiazem or verapamil, or amiodarone in the acute setting, which has the added benefit of chemically cardioverting patients to sinus rhythm. But beware the interaction with beta-blockers, leading to possible bradycardia

- There is currently no consensus on the recommendation for anticoagulation during thyroid storm

- Aggressive cooling with paracetamol, ice packs and mechanical cooling should be performed for patients with high fever

- ICU admission is recommended for all thyroid storm patients

Specific Management when FEELING LOW

Dangerously low levels of electrolytes and hormones are treated by replacement (if the low concentration isn't due to water overload, and thus haemodilution). The actual amount you give depends on the severity of depletion, the rate of depletion, and the response of the patient (Table 17.4).

Table 17.4 Managing electrolyte deficiency

	Parenteral replacement (IV)	Enteral replacement (PO/NG)
Potassium	• 40 mmol K⁺ in 1000 mL of 0.9% sodium chloride • For peripheral infusions, can be given no quicker than 10 mmol/h, which is unlikely to significantly impact on total body deficit • If rapid correction required, this can be given via central venous access and in a monitored environment such as ICU. This is normally provided in 100 mL bags containing 40 mmol K⁺, which can be given at 25–50 mL/h (i.e. up to 20 mmol/h)	• Sando K® (12 mmol/tab) • Slow-K (8 mmol/tab) NB – can cause oesophageal irritation. Tell the patient to take the tablets in an upright position, drinking water before and after
Magnesium	• 2–5 g (4–20 mmol) Mg²⁺ NB – aim for an overall plasma Mg²⁺ of 1 mmol/L	• Magnesium glycerophosphate (4 mmol/tab)
Sodium	• Complex, and rapid correction of low sodium can be catastrophic • Familiarise yourself with how many mmol/L of Na⁺ there are in all the different types of fluids available • Do not raise Na⁺ by >10 mmol/L per 24 hours and seek senior help • Hypertonic saline is sometimes used to correct severe hyponatraemia in the presence of fitting or cerebral oedema. Patients with these symptoms need urgent ICU referral	• Slow Sodium® (10 mmol/tab)
Calcium	• 10 mL of 10% calcium chloride (6.8 mmol/10 mL) Or • 10 mL of 10% calcium gluconate (2.26 mmol/10 mL)	• Calcichew® (12.6 mmol/tab) NB – there are a large number of oral calcium supplements available

	Parenteral replacement (IV)	Enteral replacement (PO/NG)

Glucose	**For hypoglycaemic coma:**
	• 50 mL of 20% glucose (IV)
	Or if no IV access:
	• 1 mg glucagon IM or SC
		Hypoglycaemia:
		• 10–20 g glucose, which is equivalent to:
		  • 2 teaspoons of sugar
		  • 1 Glucogel (Hypostop gel) ampoule
		  • 90 mL Coca-Cola

Thyroid hormone	**For hypothyroid coma:** • Liothyronine sodium 50 mcg, slow intravenous injection (then 25 mcg every 8 h) NB – remember to give a shot of steroid (100 mg hydrocortisone IV) when treating severe hypothyroidism – treating hypothyroidism can unmask life-threatening hypoadrenalism	• Levothyroxine, 50–100 mcg (then titrated up to a maintenance dose in steps of 25–50 mcg every 3–4 weeks) NB – dose reduction is required in cardiac and elderly patients
Steroid hormones/ adrenal crisis	**For acute adrenocortical insufficiency = adrenal crisis:** • Hydrocortisone 100 mg, IV/IM (then 200 mg hydrocortisone infusion/24 h) • 0.9% sodium chloride, 1000 mL within the first hour (then further intravenous rehydration – usually 4–6 L in 24 h; monitor for fluid overload in case of renal impairment and in elderly patients)	**Addison's disease/post adrenalectomy:** • Hydrocortisone 20 mg OD PO • Dose usually divided 2/3–1/3, with the larger dose given in the morning, thereby consistent with the physiological circadian rhythm of cortisol • +/– fludrocortisone 50–300 mcg PO

Practical Prescribing in General Gastroenterology

Chapter 18

Angad Singh

Gastrointestinal complaints are common. Here are some top tips to help you manage them.

Dyspepsia (Non-Ulcer)

STOP! Firstly, check that the diagnosis isn't more serious. Then, before wading in with any treatment, determine any possible cause for the dyspepsia, e.g. NSAIDs, delayed gastric emptying, caffeine intake – and then manage appropriately.

If no removable cause is present, start with a 4-week course of a PPI and then reassess the symptoms.

Reducing Stomach Acid Secretion

Table 18.1 Management of conditions caused by high gastric acid secretion

Drugs	
PPIs are the drugs of choice, e.g.:	
• omeprazole 10–40 mg OD	
• lansoprazole 15–30 mg OD	
Treatment regimens for:	
Non-ulcer dyspepsia	If no removable cause then a 4-week course of PPI, then reassess
Gastro-oesophageal reflux disease	Commence a 1–2 month course of PPI Then reduce therapy to the lowest dose that controls symptoms

(cont.)

With acknowledgement to Caroline Green and Rebecca White, who were the original authors of this chapter.

Table 18.1 *(cont.)*

Treatment regimens for:	
Duodenal ulcers	Eradicate *H. pylori*
	If ulceration is still present, continue with another 4 weeks of a PPI
	If symptoms continue, repeat the 4-week course of PPI, then reduce dose to the lowest possible that controls symptoms
Gastric ulcers	Eradicate *H. pylori*
	Continue PPI treatment for another 8 weeks
	Check endoscopy at 6–8 weeks and make a decision regarding continuing treatment
Acute GI bleed from an ulcer	Having endoscoped the patient, your gastroenterologist might ask you to prescribe a PPI infusion, i.e. omeprazole loading dose 80 mg then 8 mg/hour for 72 hours

Helicobacter pylori eradication therapy

- This is a 1-week oral course of three drugs: one PPI and two antibiotics
- The actual antibiotics will depend on local policy and penicillin allergies
- An example: omeprazole 20 mg BD, amoxicillin 1 g BD (or metronidazole 400 mg BD), clarithromycin 500 mg BD

Diarrhoea

- First, resuscitate (fluids AND electrolytes might be depleted). Try oral first if at all possible.
- Identify the cause and treat appropriately (e.g. cancer/infection/colitis). ALWAYS ensure (especially in the elderly) that this isn't faecal impaction with overflow.
- If antidiarrhoeal agents are required (ASK SOMEONE MORE SENIOR FIRST – do not use in overflow diarrhoea caused by faecal impaction, or in infective diarrhoea), use:
  - codeine phosphate 30 mg TDS or QDS PO, *or*
  - loperamide 4 mg PO initially, then 2 mg after each loose stool for up to 5 days (a maximum of 16 mg daily).

High-Output Stomas

Principles of management of high-output stoma:

- Correct dehydration with IV fluids.
- Restrict oral fluid intake, otherwise this can drive the high output stoma.
- Typically, oral fluid intake is restricted to 1.5 L, of which 500 mL is for water, juice, tea, coffees etc. and the remaining 1 L is either St. Mark's solution or double strength Dioralyte®.
- Always consult local nutrition team or gastroenterology team.
- Drugs such as loperamide, omeprazole and codeine can also be used to limit stomal losses.
- Octreotide may also be used to reduce stomal losses.

Inflammatory Bowel Disease

This is a specialist area, but here are some basics while you wait for the gastroenterology registrar to review.

Treatment of acute exacerbations (in prediagnosed patient) include:

- fluid resuscitation
- thromboprophylaxis with SC low molecular weight heparin (see Chapter 29 – Parenteral Anticoagulation)
- hydrocortisone 100 mg QDS IV, switching to oral prednisolone 40 mg after 5 days (assuming symptoms are improving), reducing by 5 mg every week until off steroids. PPI and Adcal D3® should also be prescribed for stomach and bone protection. Should symptoms not improve, a specialist gastroenterology opinion is needed.

If continuing or commencing an aminosalicylate, the precise preparation will depend on where the disease is located. Follow specialist advice.

Prescribing Pre-Endoscopy

Prescribing in patients who are on anticoagulant/antiplatelet agents and undergoing endoscopic procedures can be difficult to remember. Consult Figures 18.1 and 18.2 and if still unsure, check with the endoscopist!

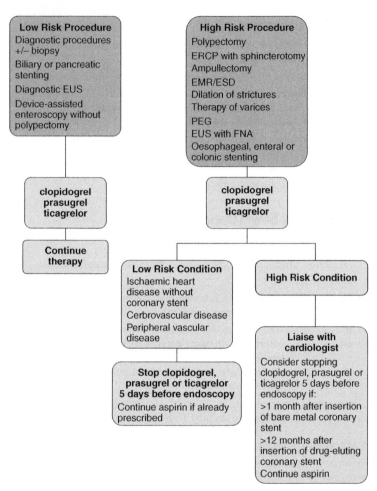

Figure 18.1 Guidelines for the management of patients on P2Y12 receptor antagonist antiplatelet agents undergoing endoscopic procedures. (From Veitch EM et al. Endoscopy in patients on antiplatelet or anticoagulant therapy, including direct oral anticoagulants: British Society of Gastroenterology (BSG) and European Society of Gastrointestinal Endoscopy (ESGE) guidelines. *Gut* 2016, 65: 374–389. Used with permission.)

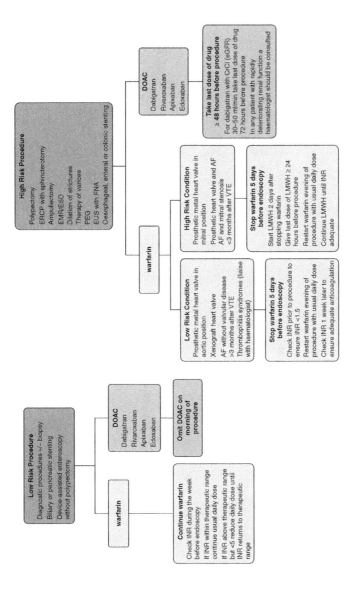

Figure 18.2 Guidelines for the management of patients on warfarin or direct oral anticoagulants (DOAC) undergoing endoscopic procedures. (From Veitch EM et al. Endoscopy in patients on antiplatelet or anticoagulant therapy, including direct oral anticoagulant therapy: British Society of Gastroenterology (BSG) and European Society of Gastrointestinal Endoscopy (ESGE) guidelines. *Gut* 2016; 65: 374–389. Used with permission.)

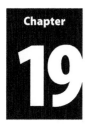

Chapter

19

Constipation in the Adult Patient

Angad Singh

A common scenario! A **DIPER** will prevent you falling between stools!

Diagnosis

What is normal for your patient – three bowel movements a day or three a week? Constipation isn't necessarily lack of frequency: it might be the passing of hard, painful faeces or difficulty in full evacuation.

Identify a Cause

Look for all the Ds:

- disease – e.g. endocrine, metabolic or neurological disturbances
- disability (immobility)
- dietary change – never underestimate the effect of hospital food
- dehydration
- drug treatment – e.g. antacids containing aluminium, anticholinergics, iron salts, opioid analgesics including co-proxamol, phenothiazines, tricyclic antidepressants, verapamil, antiparkinsonian drugs, diuretics, amiodarone, clonidine, lithium, NSAIDS and antidiarrhoeals.

Prompt the patient

Encourage your patient:

- to increase fibre intake. Rich sources include wholegrains, oats, vegetables, fruit and linseeds
- to drink enough (2 L per day)
- to exercise.

Elect to Prescribe a Laxative

NOT the first step in the management of constipation! If you have to use drugs, use the least number of drugs for the least amount of time.

With acknowledgement to Olivia Hanmeer, who was the original author of this chapter. **81**

When choosing a laxative, current NICE guidelines suggest the following approach:

- *Bulk-forming laxatives* (containing soluble fibre) act by retaining fluid within the stool and increasing faecal mass, stimulating peristalsis; also have stool-softening properties:
  - Ispaghula husk
  - Methylcellulose
  - Sterculia
- *Osmotic laxatives* act by increasing the amount of fluid in the large bowel producing distension, which leads to stimulation of peristalsis; lactulose and macrogols also have stool-softening properties.
  - Lactulose
  - Macrogols (polyethylene glycols)
  - Phosphate and sodium citrate enemas
- *Stimulant laxatives* cause peristalsis by stimulating colonic nerves (senna) or colonic and rectal nerves (bisacodyl, sodium picosulfate).
  - Senna – hydrolysed to the active metabolite by bacterial enzymes in the large bowel
  - Bisacodyl and sodium picosulfate – hydrolysed to the same active metabolite. Bisacodyl is hydrolysed by intestinal enzymes; sodium picosulfate relies on colonic bacteria
  - Docusate – a surface-wetting agent which reduces the surface tension of the stool, allowing water to penetrate and soften it. Also has a relatively weak stimulant effect.

It's also important to document when laxatives were started, as the full effect can only be seen if administered for long enough.

Other Laxatives

In recent years, newer drugs have been released for treatment of chronic constipation.

These include prucalopride, lubiprostone and linaclotide. These tend to be prescribed by gastroenterologists and typically in the setting of outpatient clinics.

Naloxegol can be used for opioid-induced constipation and continues while patients remain on opioids. CANNOT be given in conjunction with clarithromycin.

Review the patient

Stool charts should be kept. A fluid balance chart is also helpful. Review laxative therapy regularly and discontinue when no longer needed. Laxative dependence should be avoided.

Chapter 20

Nausea and Vomiting

Angad Singh

Choose an antiemetic according to the mechanism of vomiting (Table 20.1). Is the cause of nausea central, vestibular, toxin-related or due to gastric outflow obstruction? Imagine you have gone out for a heavy night's drinking …

You drink 10 pints in a couple of hours. You feel sick, have a large volume vomit and feel better. Mechanism of vomiting: gastric distension. You need a PROKINETIC, e.g. metoclopramide or domperidone.

Avoiding beers this time! You drink shots all night. Less volume. At the end of the night you feel sick. Mechanism of nausea: poisoning. You need a CENTRALLY ACTING drug, e.g. haloperidol (D_2 antagonist) or cyclizine (H_2 antagonist and anticholinergic).

Table 20.1 Antiemetics

Drug	Mechanism of action	Clinical uses
Metoclopramide	Prokinetic, weak D_2 antagonist	Gastric outflow obstruction Upper GI bleed Liver metastases Cancer head of pancreas
Haloperidol	Not just for sedating delirious older patients Good central antiemetic effect (D_2 antagonist)	Poisoning related nausea Hypercalcaemia Uraemia, antibiotics, opioids
Cyclizine	ACh/H_2 (central acting)	Raised intracranial pressure Central causes Motion sickness/vestibular problems
Ondansetron/ Granisetron	$5HT_3$ antagonist	Chemo-induced nausea

With acknowledgement to Simon Noble and Clare Turner, who were the original authors of this chapter.

You finally settle. Friends get you into a taxi. You are sick. Mechanism: vestibular disturbance. You need something to work on the acetylcholine/H_2 receptors (cyclizine or prochlorperazine).

Top TIPS for Treating Nausea

- Ondansetron only hits one receptor. What's more it constipates you!
- Haloperidol and cyclizine make a good combination, covering many receptors.
- NEVER give metoclopramide and cyclizine together. The antimuscarinic effect of cyclizine blocks the prokinetic effect of metoclopramide rendering it as much help as a chocolate fireguard.
- The 'Domestos' of antiemetics is levomepromazine. The reason it is not regularly used is because it is sedating. It's best to talk to the palliative care team before using it (see Chapter 27 – Palliative Care Prescribing).

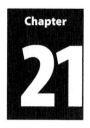

Safe Prescribing in Liver Disease
Angad Singh

Drugs Commonly Used/Seen in Liver Disease

Spironolactone
Used in the management of ascites. Mechanism of action means it takes 72 hours to have an effect so do not increase dose if already increased within 72 hours. Patients usually start on 100 mg daily, increasing to a maximum dose of 400 mg. Main side effects include electrolyte disturbance (hyponatraemia, hyperkalaemia) and gynaecomastia.

Furosemide
Often used in combination with spironolactone, often starting at 40 mg daily. Can be increased in stepwise progression to maximum of 160 mg OD. Main side effects are related to electrolyte disturbance (hyponatraemia, hypokalaemia).

Ciprofloxacin
Patients who have had an episode of spontaneous bacterial peritonitis are given ciprofloxacin as prophylaxis against future episodes.

Rifaximin
Prevention of encephalopathy in patients who have had a previous episode of encephalopathy. Dose 550 mg BD.

Propanolol/Carvedilol
Used in patients with varices, either as primary or secondary prophylaxis, to minimise the risk of variceal haemorrhage by reducing portal pressure.

With acknowledgement to Caroline Green and Rebecca White, who were the original authors of this chapter.

Lactulose

Treatment with lactulose is based on the absence of a specific disaccharidase on the microvillus membrane of enterocytes in the human small bowel, thereby permitting entry of the disaccharides into the colon.

In the colon, lactulose is catabolised by the bacterial flora to short chain fatty acids (e.g. lactic acid and acetic acid), which lower the colonic pH to approximately 5. The reduction in pH favours the formation of the non-absorbable NH_4^+ from NH_3, trapping NH_4^+ in the colon and thus reducing plasma ammonia concentrations.

Terlipressin

Indications:

- Variceal bleed (1 mg QDS for 5 days)
- Hepatorenal syndrome (0.5 mg–2 mg for up to 2 weeks).

Use in caution with patients with known ischaemic heart disease, cardiac arrythmias and contraindicated in pregnancy.

Drugs to Avoid
NSAIDs

Non-steroidal anti-inflammatory drugs should not be used in patients with ascites because of the high risk of developing further sodium retention, hyponatraemia and AKI.

ACEi

Angiotensin converting enzyme inhibitors, angiotensin II antagonists or α1-adrenergic receptor blockers should not generally be used in patients with ascites because of the increased risk of renal impairment.

Aminoglycoside Antibiotics e.g. Gentamicin

Avoid if possible due to risk of renal impairment.

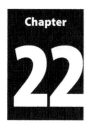

Chapter 22

Practical Parenteral Nutrition

Laura Coughlan and Angad Singh

Two Golden Facts

- One-third of people aged 65 years or over are at risk of malnutrition on admission to hospital.
- Malnutrition kills – but in ways you won't spot (it affects every system in the body and results in increased susceptibility to illness and infections).

So feed your patients!

Two Golden Rules

- Involve the dietitian EARLY – as soon as you suspect malnutrition or the risk of malnutrition.
- If the gut works, use it! If the patient cannot swallow, place a fine-bore feeding tube: this can be done at the bedside and placement is confirmed by checking pH. If unsuccessful then an X-ray is required, which only an FY2 and above can interpret.

What About Parenteral Nutrition?

Seek advice from your nutrition team! Commonly, you will just be asked to sign the prescription. Before putting pen to paper, think **SICKLy** – you need to **KNOW**…

- The indication for PN? Remember: PN is never an emergency (except in children). Indications for PN include prolonged ileus, short bowel syndrome, gastrointestinal obstruction (where enteral feeding isn't possible), complex fistulae and severe malabsorption.
- Low albumin does not indicate that the patient is malnourished: it is usually an indicator of how sick they are. PN is not a cure for low albumin. Inflammation reduces albumin levels due to an increase in cytokines resulting in a raised CRP (meaning other proteins like albumin are not proritised for production in the liver).

- What is the goal of PN and expected duration? If home PN is required a referral to a tertiary centre will be needed.
- Recent biochemistry, including Ca^{2+}, Mg^{2+}, PO_4^{2-}, K^+, Na^+.
- A recent weight? Has there been unintentional weight loss?
- Has a fluid restriction been set? Or are there high GI losses that need replacing?
- What venous access do they have/require for PN? Dedicated access is required.

Then, KNOW What's in a Bag and How Much

Dietitian and pharmacist will calculate:

- Calories as glucose and fat
- Protein as basic amino acids (expressed as grams of nitrogen)
- Water
- Electrolytes – Na^+, K^+, Ca^{2+}, Mg^{2+}, PO_4^{2-}
- Vitamins and trace elements (do not check trace elements when CRP ↑ as levels can be falsely ↓).

Dietitians use standard equations to predict energy requirements. These are based on clinical condition, age, weight, body mass index and physical activity levels. Estimated requirements are altered for obese patients and estimated dry weights are used when oedema/ascites is present. Different equations are used for intubated patients.

REMEMBER: more isn't better! Overfeeding is the cause of most complications.

Other complications include:

- Overhydration/oedema – ensure excess IV fluids are not prescribed
- Hyperglycemia – blood glucose levels should be checked regularly. If continued high levels, consider insulin
- Electrolyte abnormalities (see below)
- Deranged liver function tests (mostly this is not due to PN and other factors need to be considered, e.g. sepsis, medications, underlying liver disease. Can consider looking at fat provision in PN or commence cyclical feeding)
- Hypertriglyceridaemia – monitor levels if high, consider taking lipid out of bag for a short period.

Lastly, KNOW About Refeeding Syndrome in Sick, Malnourished Patients

Here, a surge in insulin levels causes a rapid drop in K^+, PO_4^{2-}, Mg^{2+} and Ca^{2+} levels, which can have severe clinical consequences. Avoid by starting at a low rate and build up, monitor electrolytes daily, supplementing as required. Prescribe Pabrinex ampoules 1 and 2 OD for 48 hours.

Chapter

Analgesia

Suparna Bali

(See also, Chapter 27 – Palliative Care Prescribing)

Poor analgesic control will diminish a patient's quality of life and may slow hospital recovery, as will treatment with the wrong doses or combinations of drugs! The following will make your life easier:

a. Understanding the concepts of basic analgesia

b. Getting advice *early*!

c. Engaging your hospital's 'Pain Team'.

		Step 3 Opioid (strong) for moderate to severe pain, e.g. morphine +/– non-opioid
	Step 2 Opioid (weak) for mild to moderate pain +/– non-opioid	
Step 1 Non-opioid, e.g. paracetamol +/or NSAID		

Figure 23.1 The World Health Organization (WHO) Analgesic Ladder. (Data from: www.who.int/cancer/palliative/painladder/en.)

TOP TIPS Using the Analgesic Ladder (Figure 23.1)

- Start at the bottom 'rung' with paracetamol or NSAIDs. If ineffective, use both together.

- If this fails, move up the ladder – DO NOT add another from the same class!

- Regular administration of analgesia is more effective than 'PRN' dosing; total drug administered with regular dosing will also be lower than PRN.

(cont.)

- Whatever drug you choose, start with the lowest possible dose, then increase according to response (which will differ from patient to patient).
- Avoid the use of more than one opioid at a time.
- The ladder has no top 'rung' as there is no upper limit for strong opioids. However, if high doses are being used then the cause of the pain must be reinvestigated.

Table 23.1 shows examples of step 1 and 2 drugs: their usual doses, routes of administration, and some advantages and disadvantages of their use. However, you may come across patients who fall outside these general prescribing rules. For example, codeine does not work in around 10% of the population as they lack the enzyme to break it down to an opioid. In contrast, those with renal impairment are unable to excrete the drug effectively and will develop side effects much more quickly. Therefore, efficacy and side effects are *highly variable* and should be watched for.

NSAIDs (Based on MHRA Safety Advice December 2014)

Base your choice on an assessment of a patient's individual risk factors, including any history of cardiovascular disease and the relative gastrointestinal safety, tolerability and efficacy relevant to your patient's clinical situation. The risk of cardiovascular disease and gastrointestinal toxicity is higher in the elderly population. Naproxen and low-dose ibuprofen are considered to have the most favourable thrombotic cardiovascular safety profiles of all non-selective NSAIDs.

Never use more than one NSAID at a time.

RED ALERT: NSAIDs

Before prescribing NSAIDs check for:

- Hypersensitivity and allergic reactions to aspirin or NSAIDs
- Asthma
- History of cardiovascular disease
- History of peptic ulcer disease or GI bleed
- Renal impairment
- Liver impairment
- Coagulopathy.

Table 23.1 WHO Analgesic Ladder: Steps 1 and 2

Drug	Dose	Plus points	Down side
Non-opioids			
Paracetamol	1 g QDS	Can be given PO, PR and IV. Intravenous has a rapid onset of action (5 minutes) Not known to be harmful in pregnancy	*Caution in severe liver/renal disease Do not use in acute liver failure* Increased risk of toxicity (at therapeutic doses) especially in body weight <50 kg and those with risk factors for hepatotoxicity. Dose adjustment required No anti-inflammatory effect
Ibuprofen (NSAID)	1.2 g–1.8 g in three to four divided doses PO. Can be increased to a max. 2.4 g daily	Anti-inflammatory Analgesic and antipyretic effects Topical preparation available	*Avoid in:* • Liver disease • Renal disease • Those with a history of peptic ulcer disease *Caution in:* • Asthma • Concurrent anticoagulation • Inflammatory bowel disease
Diclofenac sodium[a] (NSAID)	75–150 mg in divided doses PO or PR (max. 150 mg/24 h) Can be given deep IM but only for 2 days	As for ibuprofen Can be given PO, PR and IV Topical preparation available	As for ibuprofen Contraindicated in patients with established: • Ischaemic heart disease • Peripheral arterial disease • Cerebrovascular disease • Congestive heart failure

(cont.)

Table 23.1 (cont.)

Drug	Dose	Plus points	Down side
Opioids			
Codeine[b]	30–60 mg every 4–6 hours PO or 30–60 mg every 4 hours IM	For mild to moderate pain	*Caution* in renal/liver impairment Will not work for 10% of patients due to enzyme deficiency Can cause constipation
Dihydrocodeine	30 mg every 4–6 hours PO or up to 50 mg deep SC 4–6 hourly	Analgesic efficacy similar to codeine	*Caution* in renal/liver impairment Can cause constipation Greater incidence of nausea than codeine
Tramadol[c]	50–100 mg every 4–6 hours PO, IM or IV	Acts at serotonergic receptors as well as opiate receptors so useful for neuropathic pain Less constipating than codeine	*Caution* in renal/liver impairment Contraindicated in uncontrolled epilepsy Can cause hallucinations

[a] See safety reminder (a) below.
[b] See safety reminder (b) below.
[c] See safety reminder (c) below.
For further information consult manufacturers' product characteristics.

Safety Reminders (Table 23.1)

a. Diclofenac is now contraindicated in patients with established ischaemic heart disease, peripheral arterial disease, cerebrovascular disease and congestive heart failure. Diclofenac treatment should only be initiated after careful consideration for patients with significant risk factors for cardiovascular events (e.g. hypertension, hyperlipidaemia, diabetes mellitus, smoking).

b. As codeine is metabolised to morphine, important safety information from the MHRA from July 2013 advised that it should only be used in children >12 years and only where pain cannot be relieved by other painkillers like paracetamol or ibuprofen due to reports of morphine toxicity. Codeine is contraindicated in patients of any age who are known to be ultra-rapid metabolisers of codeine.

c. Tramadol is a schedule 3 controlled drug (since June 2014) hence 'controlled drug' prescription requirements apply.

Compound Analgesics

Compound analgesics, used for mild to moderate pain, contain paracetamol (or aspirin) combined with an opioid (e.g. codeine, dihydrocodeine).

Table 23.2 indicates the content of one tablet (expressed in proportions of x/y strengths in milligrams) of each of the common preparations.

Table 23.2 Tablet contents of common compound analgesics

Compound analgesic	Content of one tablet
Co-codamol 8/500	Codeine phosphate 8 mg and paracetamol 500 mg
Co-codamol 30/500 (Solpadol®, Tylex®)	Codeine phosphate 30 mg and paracetamol 500 mg
Co-dydramol 10/500	Dihydrocodeine 10 mg and paracetamol 500 mg

RED ALERT: Paracetamol

The maximum dose of paracetamol is 1 g QDS: check this is not being exceeded with these compound preparations. Always check when paracetamol was last administered. Susceptible groups (e.g. the elderly) will be at risk of side effects even with the low dose opioid in these compound preparations.

Although useful to encourage compliance in chronic pain conditions, such compound preparations will not allow you to titrate the doses of the constituent drugs separately. This may hamper optimal acute pain management.

Opioid Analgesics

Opioids offer valuable analgesia for moderate to severe pain. Opioids can be administered by different routes and their use should be tailored to the patient's needs. This can be achieved by the regular prescribing of modified release opioids (every 12 hours) with immediate release preparations available for 'breakthrough' pain offering pain relief around the clock.

The idea that 'morphine derivatives' are only reserved for cancer patients is wrong! Yes, there are potential side effects (nausea, vomiting, drowsiness, constipation, pruritis, tolerance and addiction) and large doses can cause respiratory depression and hypotension. However, this should not deter from prescribing them where appropriate.

Opioids should generally be prescribed for short courses, to minimise the risk of addiction. Table 23.3 shows the opioid conversion table (BNF 74).

Table 23.3 Opioid conversion table (BNF 74)

Drug	Dose	Route	Approx. equivalent oral morphine dose
Codeine	100 mg	PO	10 mg
Dihydrocodeine	100 mg	PO	10 mg
Diamorphine	3 mg	SC/IM/IV	10 mg
Hydromorphone	2 mg	PO	10 mg
Morphine sulfate (immediate release)	10 mg	PO	10 mg
Morphine sulfate	5 mg	SC/IM/IV	10 mg
Oxycodone	6.6 mg	PO	10 mg
Tramadol	100 mg	PO	10 mg

NB – These are approximate conversions; other reference sources may differ

TOP TIPS When Prescribing Opioids

- Prescribe an antiemetic *prophylactically*, e.g. cyclizine 50 mg TDS to pre-empt nausea
- Prescribe a laxative e.g. senna two tablets nocte
- Pruritis may be relieved by an antihistamine, e.g. chlorphenamine
- Patients can develop tolerance to opioids: you may need to increase doses with prolonged use
- Naloxone 0.4–2 mg every 2–3 mins IV/SC/IM (max. 10 mg – seek specialist advice) will reverse opioid effects, thereby useful if respiratory depression or hypotension ensue. But remember that the half-life of naloxone is very short, so with long half-life opioids, e.g. methadone, you may have to give repeated doses
- Naloxone is also a good diagnostic tool whenever opioid toxicity/abuse is suspected. Naloxone should wake the patient up for seconds, before the patient reverts to their original state. If respiratory function does not improve then question the diagnosis.

Remember

When converting a patient from regular oral morphine sulfate (immediate release) to morphine sulfate (modified release):

- Add up the total amount of morphine administered in 24 hours (including PRN doses)
- Halve this amount to give a twice daily (BD) morphine modified-release dose
- e.g. 10 mg QDS immediate release morphine = 40 mg in 24 hours = *20 mg BD modified release morphine.*

Transdermal Fentanyl (Refer to Product Monograph and Seek Specialist Advice)

The initial fentanyl patch dose should be based on the patient's previous opioid history, including the degree of opioid tolerance, if any. Patches must be replaced every 72 hours.

A recommended conversion scheme (adapted from the BNF) for oral morphine to a fentanyl patch is given in Table 23.4. As conversion ratios vary, these figures are a guide only.

The initial evaluation of the analgesic effect of the transdermal fentanyl should not be made before the patch has been worn for 24 hours due to the gradual increase in serum fentanyl concentrations up to this time. Previous analgesic therapy should therefore be phased out gradually from the time of first application of the patch until analgesic efficacy with fentanyl is attained. Additional breakthrough doses of analgesia may still be required on continuation of patch.

Remember – fentanyl levels fall gradually once the patch is removed, taking up to 20 hours or more for the fentanyl serum concentration to decrease by 50%.

Table 23.4 Conversion scheme for oral morphine to a fentanyl patch

Oral 24-hour morphine salt (mg/day)	Transdermal fentanyl dose (mcg/h)
30	12
60	25
120	50
180	75
240	100

Patient-Controlled Analgesia

Suparna Bali

What is PCA?

'Patient-controlled analgesia' (PCA) is used for the control of moderate to severe pain in the acute postoperative period. It allows patients to self-administer preprogrammed small boluses of IV or SC opioids, e.g. morphine, at the push of a button (a 'successful demand' by the patient). A lock-out time is also programmed during which a repeat dose cannot be delivered even if requested (unsuccessful demands). Often, a background infusion rate is also prescribed.

Advantages include:

- Fewer adverse effects and faster recovery time
- No repeated intramuscular or subcutaneous injections
- Avoids the 'peaks and troughs' of opioid levels
- Patient empowerment through improved analgesia (patient can titrate to effect)
- Reduced patient anxiety
- Less nursing time.

Remember – Take into account the number of times the patient has 'demanded' (self-administered) a PCA bolus since commencement. A high number of unsuccessful demands by the patient may indicate either a lack of understanding of how the PCA works or inadequate pain relief.

RED ALERT: ALWAYS Check Patient Suitability for PCAs

Contraindications include:

- Patient refusal
- Inability to comprehend PCA concept (e.g. confused/drowsy patient)
- Reduced dexterity, e.g. arthritis, burns
- Where opioids are contraindicated
- Untrained medical/nursing staff.

TOP TIPS for PCAs

1. Ongoing education of the patient (starting preoperatively) about the PCA is paramount:
   - Tell them how the machine works
   - Reassure about minimal risk of opioid addiction or overdose
   - Explain that they must 'keep pain away' by pressing the button before the pain becomes severe.

2. A PCA prescription should generally include:
   - The name and total amount of drug required
   - The name and amount of diluent required
   - Route of administration
   - The final drug concentration
   - The PCA bolus dose
   - The lock-out period
   - Naloxone (so that the effect of overdosed opioid can be rapidly reversed)
   - Details of any continuous background infusion that may be required.

Remember – The patient usually comes back from theatre with a PCA already prescribed by the anaesthetist. This may be on a special proforma – *always double-check.*

Chapter 25

Epidural Analgesia
Suparna Bali

Epidural analgesia is safe and effective in providing pain relief before, during and after a surgical procedure (thoracic, abdominal, obstetric and hip surgery) or in the management of chronic pain. In general, small quantities of local anaesthetic and opioid analgesic agents are used in combination and administered by slow infusion into the epidural space. Doses used (and therefore side effects) are far less than would be required with systemic administration. Therefore, epidurals can reduce the likelihood of complications such as chest infection, DVT and pressure sores.

RED ALERT: Contraindications for Epidural Analgesia

- Patient refusal
- Bleeding disorders (including concurrent anticoagulant therapy; *caution* with NSAIDs)
- Infection/bacteraemia (risk of epidural abscess)
- Active local infection of skin at epidural site
- Hypovolaemia or hypotension
- Raised intracranial pressure
- Allergy to drug(s) used
- Spinal disorder (relative contraindication).

Choice of Opioid
Fentanyl is a common option in epidurals: its high lipid solubility means it has a rapid onset of action as it passes through the CSF quickly. It is also less likely to cause central respiratory depression, as it is easily absorbed by local nerve tissue.

Choice of Local Anaesthetic

Local anaesthetic (LA) causes a reversible block to nerve conduction, depending on the strength of the LA as well as the size of the nerve. The stronger the LA used in epidurals the more likely they are to block motor as well as sensory function. Hence, weak solutions, e.g. bupivacaine 0.125%, can provide good analgesia with minimal motor impairment. Both types of block should be checked routinely.

Complications of Epidural Anaesthesia

Patients may come back to you from theatre with an epidural already in situ and prescribed on a special proforma. Your job is to look out for the potential complications and alert the anaesthetist. Here are some examples:

- *Hypotension and bradycardia:* Due to sympathetic blockade by the local anaesthetic. Reduce rate or stop epidural and review effect. Once haemorrhage, fluid depletion or inappropriately high epidural block has been excluded, treat with a fluid bolus and/or ephedrine.

- *Catheter migration:* The epidural catheter can accidentally migrate from the epidural space to the subarachnoid space where the opioid is more concentrated than required for a spinal block. Thus the patient receives an excessive dose which can lead to increased analgesia, sedation and respiratory depression.

- *Dural puncture headache:* If this occurs, treat the symptoms and ensure adequate hydration. The patient must avoid straining, e.g. treat constipation.

- *Epidural haematoma:* Unintentional damage to an epidural blood vessel can cause bleeding into the epidural space resulting in pressure on the spinal cord; always routinely check the patient's motor (assessing myotomes) and sensory function (assessing dermatomes using an ethyl chloride spray or ice cube, where the dermatome at which sensation returns correlates to the level of the block: remember, pain and temperature are carried in the same spinal tract).

- *Local anaesthetic toxicity:* One of the initial symptoms is a 'tingling' sensation round the mouth which, if not identified quickly, can lead to more serious consequences, including convulsions, coma and cardiac arrest. If this is suspected, stop the epidural immediately and contact the anaesthetists/pain team urgently, as administration of intralipid may be warranted.

- *Epidural abscess:* Infection can develop at the site of the epidural placement and develop into an abscess. Prolonged catheterisation can increase the risk of this occurring.

TOP TIPS When Prescribing Epidurals

- Most hospitals have a separate epidural chart (check first) which should include the maximum and minimum rate for the infusion.

- The patient's drug chart must *clearly indicate* that the patient is receiving an epidural infusion.

- Concurrent opioids should only be prescribed *on advice of the pain/anaesthetic team*.

- Pre-empt side effects associated with opioids and LAs by prescribing antiemetics, laxatives, antihistamines and naloxone.

- Check your hospital guidelines for the INR range within which the epidural catheter can be removed (usually between 1 and 1.5).

- Remember that an epidural catheter can only be sited 12 hours after a prophylactic dose of LMWH or 24 hours after a treatment dose, and that LMWH can only be administered 4 hours following its removal.

- Be aware of any prescribed medication which may affect clotting, e.g. heparins, antiplatelets or anticoagulants.

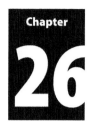

Chapter 26

Fit for a Fit: How to Treat Adults with Seizures

Lindsey Stockford and
Sheetal Sumaria

What to do if my patient is fitting? When should I get concerned and intervene?

In general, don't treat the first unprovoked seizure as there is no evidence this will affect the long-term prognosis.

However, if a patient is having a convulsion lasting longer than 5 minutes, or they have had two convulsions without full recovery of consciousness in between ('status epilepticus by definition'), it is time to crack on with treatment.

Remember, though, that you do need a good history:

• Is the patient a known epileptic?
• Is s/he taking antiepileptic medication?
• What is the seizure frequency and how long do they normally last?
• Is the patient diabetic, pregnant, a known alcoholic or all of the above?
• Are there likely to be precipitants? Fit thresholds can be lowered by drugs (e.g. haloperidol) or infection; some drugs (in toxicity) cause fits; illness may have prevented them taking their normal medicine (e.g. surgery!); other drugs might have increased the metabolism/altered the binding of their anticonvulsants.

Make sure you send blood for further investigations once you have IV access; urea and electrolytes, magnesium, calcium, liver function tests, full blood count, glucose, anticonvulsant levels and toxicology (if cause is unknown).

Despite all of this, seizure treatment is pretty much standardised.

Early Stage
Benzodiazepines

After 5 minutes of ongoing generalised convulsive seizure activity. The first-line treatment is benzodiazepine therapy (see Table 26.1).

If IV access is available and the patient is in a hospital setting, give IV lorazepam (best, as shorter acting and limited tissue loading) or diazepam.

With acknowledgement to Jane Ng, who was the original author of this chapter.

Table 26.1 Benzodiazepine treatment for seizures

Drug	Route of administration	Dose	Top tip
Lorazepam	IV slow bolus into large vein	2–4 mg	Give over 3–5 minutes Rapid administration increases risk of respiratory depression and hypotension Lorazepam injection is stored in the fridge Dose can be repeated after 5 minutes
Diazepam emulsion	IV bolus maximum 5 mg/min	5–10 mg	Dose can be repeated after 5–10 minutes
Diazepam	Rectal	Usual dose is 10 mg (consider reducing dose to 5 mg in the elderly or patients weighing less than 50 kg)	Half dose in the elderly Diazepam rectal tubes – strengths of 5 mg and 10 mg
Midazolam	Buccal	10 mg	Squirt the dose onto the buccal mucosa in the mouth This is a schedule 3 controlled drug – it will be stored in a CD cupboard Unlicensed use in adult patients Dose can be repeated after 10 minutes.

REPEAT benzodiazepine dose if seizure is not terminated (see Table 26.1 for dosing interval).

If no IV access is possible or the patient is not in a hospital setting, rectal diazepam or buccal midazolam are alternatives. NB: a dose of buccal midazolam can be repeated if the seizure is not terminated 10 minutes after the first dose.

RED ALERT: When Giving Benzodiazepines

- Carefully monitor respiratory rate and blood pressure, especially when administered IV.
- Diazepam injections cause thrombophlebitis – always use Diazemuls®.
- Take special care in the elderly → reduce dose.

If the seizure has not been aborted after about 20 minutes, there is incomplete recovery between fits, there is marked hypoxia associated with the fits or if there are other worrying factors (haemodynamics compromise/associated head or neck injury suspected), CALL AN ANAESTHETIST OR ICU STAFF TO HELP; roll up your sleeves and get ready for the next step below.

Established Status Epilepticus

After 20 minutes of generalised convulsive seizures despite benzodiazepine treatment, a second-line antiepileptic should be administered (IV levetiracetam, IV sodium valproate or IV phenytoin). There is no evidence that there is any difference in efficacy between levetiracetam, sodium valproate or phenytoin. Therefore, the choice of antiepileptic should be made based on patient suitability, e.g. gender, age and reproductive status.

Levetiracetam:

- Dose: 2 g over 15 minutes can be given in 100 mL (NaCl 0.9% or glucose 5%)
- Please note this is an unlicensed indication. Higher doses may be used in some centres.

Sodium valproate:

- Dose: 40 mg/kg (maximum dose 2.8 g) over 10 minutes. The injection is available in a 400 mg vial. This is an unlicensed indication.
- Sodium valproate should be avoided, where possible, in women of childbearing age, liver disease, mitochondrial disease, urea cycle disorders and porphyria.

Phenytoin:

- Dose: 20 mg/kg, see top tips box for administration details. Phenytoin should be avoided where possible in patients with a cardiac history or in elderly patients, due to increased risk of cardiovascular complications
- Phenytoin interacts with many medicines such as warfarin, therefore caution should be used
- Do not use in patients already taking phenytoin unless you know their plasma levels. Phenytoin levels can increase quickly due to its 'zero-order kinetics'.

TOP TIPS for Phenytoin Administration

- Dose: 20 mg/kg; a standard 1 g loading dose is suitable for most patients, but you should calculate the dose for tiny and very big patients.
- Maximum rate 50 mg/min → 1 g loading dose must be given over a minimum of 20 minutes (give undiluted via syringe pump).
- Alternatively, dilute in 100 mL of sodium chloride 0.9% and infuse over a minimum of 20 minutes using an infusion pump.

RED ALERT: When Giving Phenytoin

- Always use an inline filter (0.2–0.5 micron) when administering diluted phenytoin
- Administer via a large vein (phenytoin is very irritant)
- ECG monitoring is required for IV phenytoin loading doses
- Causes further respiratory depression
- Never give phenytoin IM.

If, despite all these valiant efforts, your patient is still fitting, you need the help of an anaesthetist/neurologist/intensivist. By the way, your patient should be on the ICU by now …

Chapter 27

Palliative Care Prescribing

Simon Noble

(See also Chapter 23 – Analgesia.)

There is no second chance to improve the quality of life of a dying patient. Getting it right allows a good death and helps lead to an uncomplicated bereavement for the family. However, there is much more to palliative care than just instituting a syringe driver. Liaise early with your palliative care team.

TOP TIPS for Opioids in Palliation

All the principles of opioid use apply here (see Chapter 23). In addition:
- Prescribe a regular antiemetic to prevent opioid-induced nausea (haloperidol can help in this regard, although generally not thought of as antiemetic!)
- Opioid-induced constipation can be very uncomfortable for patients. Always, ALWAYS, ALWAYS prescribe a regular laxative to prevent this complication. They will need a softener and a pusher, e.g. lactulose/senna (see Chapter 19 – Constipation in the Adult Patient).
- Profound constipation secondary to high doses of opioid will probably need something more potent, e.g. sodium docusate 100 mg PO TDS.
- Do not prescribe a fentanyl patch first line for someone with unstable cancer pain: its pharmacokinetics does not allow titration to acute pain.

Is the Patient Opioid Toxic?

Why is it that when a patient has a sodium level of 120 mmol/L, brain metastases and a urinary tract infection, doctors still blame the confusion on the morphine?! Think of opioids, sure – but don't become blinded by the opioid light!

Features of opioid toxicity:
- Myoclonus/metabolic flap (like the liver flap)
- Classic visual hallucinations. They tend to see dark spots in the periphery of their vision. Many people think they have seen cats, dogs or rats run under the bed. You have to ask them specifically about this – it is rarely volunteered as patients may be apprehensive of being labelled mentally unwell

(cont.)

- Drowsiness (severe toxicity)
- Respiratory depression (severe toxicity).

NOTE!

Small or 'pin-point' pupils are a sign of opioid *therapy* NOT opioid *toxicity*. You are just as likely to have small pupils from taking a couple of co-codamol tablets.

Important Calculations

Breakthrough dose of morphine:

Total dose of morphine in 24 hours divided by 6.

For example, someone on MST 60 mg BD:

$$60 \text{ mg} \times 2 = 120 \text{ mg (the total 24-hour dose)}$$

$$\text{Breakthrough dose} = (60 \text{ mg} \times 2)/6$$

$$= 120 \text{ mg}/6$$

$$= 20 \text{ mg PRN}$$

Converting Oral Morphine to SC Diamorphine via Syringe Driver

Take total 24-hour dose of morphine and divide by 3 (SC diamorphine is three times as potent as oral morphine).

For example, someone on MST 60 mg BD:

$$\text{SC diamorphine dose} = (60 \text{ mg} \times 2)/3$$

$$= 40 \text{ mg diamorphine SC over 24 hours}$$

Antiemetics and Palliation

(See Chapter 20 – Nausea and Vomiting.)

Again, all the general principles of nausea and vomiting treatment apply here. Some specifics to palliative care:

- You may well be using more ondansetron or granisetron as patients will be receiving palliative chemotherapy.
- The degree of nausea or vomiting might be more profound due to toxic drug doses, toxic drugs or disease. Another weapon available to you is *levomepromazine* (aka Nozinan), the 'domestos' of all antiemetics, 12.5– 50 mg PO every 4–8 hours, 12.5–25 mg every 6–8-hourly IV, or SC syringe driver. The reason it is not regularly used is because it is sedating. It's best to talk to the palliative care team before using it.

Syringe Drivers

Syringe drivers are not just for dying patients, though some may associate them with this purpose. They have several important indications:

- Patient unable to swallow/too ill to take medicines PO
- Patient nauseated (you try and take oral antiemetics when you're feeling sick!)
- Poor absorption, e.g. bowel stasis, pancreatic dysfunction, hypoalbuminaemia.

Note that syringe drivers in the palliative care setting are given SC. Try having an IM injection and decide which you would prefer!

Syringe drivers can be used for control of pain, nausea, restlessness and colic amongst other things. It is important that, when combinations are used, drugs mixed are compatible and do not crystallise. The following commonly used drugs can be mixed together in a syringe driver. It is unusual to mix more than three drugs together. If you need to use more than three, you should be chatting to the palliative care team or setting up a separate driver:

- Diamorphine
- Haloperidol
- Hyoscine hydrobromide
- Midazolam
- Levomepromazine
- Metoclopramide
- Cyclizine (can crystallise in saline, use water for injection) (Maximum concentration cyclizine 10 mg/mL with diamorphine 50 mg/mL.)

A useful website for checking drug compatibilities in syringe drivers is www.palliativedrugs.com and is well worth checking out. Alternatively, refer to an IV injectables guide that gives you the concentrations the drugs are available in and their compatibility.

Care in the Last 48 Hours of Life

Once the team has recognised a patient is dying, the following should be done:

- Stop all unnecessary medicines
- Ensure you write up PRN medicines for all symptomatic eventualities:
  - Pain: SC diamorphine PRN
  - Agitation: SC midazolam PRN
  - 'Death rattle' of retained secretions: SC hyoscine hydrobromide PRN
  - Nausea: SC cyclizine PRN
- If patient is on regular analgesics/antiemetics convert to syringe driver
- Communicate regularly with family.

Chapter

Warfarin Prescribing

Bridget Coleman

Warfarin is highly effective at killing rats. In the hands of the uneducated, it is just as effective at killing humans. So, here's some tips to get it right every time …

Starting Treatment with Warfarin

Speedy Anticoagulation

e.g. DVT, PE, mechanical heart valve.

Days 1 and 2: Start warfarin along with heparin/low molecular weight heparin (see Chapter 29 – Parenteral Anticoagulation). Use a baseline loading dose of 8 mg daily, individualised for the person as follows:

Factors that increase bleeding risk: subtract 1 mg from daily loading dose for each factor:

- Age >70 years (subtract 2 mg if age >80 years)
- Weight <50 kg
- Concurrent drug administration which increases effect of warfarin (check BNF if unsure)
- Significant hepatic impairment
- Renal failure with significant uraemia
- Severe anaemia and/or thrombocytopenia
- Significant cardiac failure
- Uncontrolled hyperthyroidism.

For example: if the patient weighs 45 kg (−1 mg) and is 70 years old (−1 mg) then a loading regimen of 6 mg OD should be used.

Factors that decrease warfarin effect: add 1 mg to daily dose for each factor:

- Concurrent drug treatment that decreases effect of warfarin (check BNF if unsure)

- Significant malabsorption
- Uncontrolled hypothyroidism.

For example: if the patient is taking rifampicin (+1 mg) then a loading regimen of 9 mg OD should be used

If >10 mg is required, seek expert advice.

Day 3: Take daily INRs until they stabilise and a maintenance dose is established.

Your hospital will have a nomogram to guide you through the initial dose adjustments from day 3 onwards. As these differ from place to place, check your local clinical guideline

If in doubt, seek expert advice!

Whatever your plan, all patients should receive heparin for at least 4 days. Heparin should not be discontinued until the INR stays within the therapeutic range for at least 2 days.

Less Speedy Anticoagulation

e.g. outpatients, AF.

Days 1–5: Give 5 mg OD

In those who have an increased bleeding risk (see above) give 3 mg daily.

Day 6: Return for INR: adjust dose according to nomogram.

RED ALERT

- Take a baseline INR before treatment.
- Very high INRs can be produced in sensitive patients.
- Patients with protein C and protein S deficiency risk warfarin-induced skin necrosis if anticoagulation is excessive (areas of fat: breast, buttock, thigh).

Adjusting the Dose of Warfarin in the Longer Term

Adjusting the dose can be more of an art than a science, aiming to get the INR within 0.5 either way of the target. In practice, short-term deviation by up to ± 0.75 units is acceptable, e.g. for a target INR of 2.5, anywhere between 1.75 and 3.25 is usually acceptable.

The target to aim for depends upon the reason for anticoagulation. National guidelines are being rewritten – and target INRs might end up being reduced for AF in the elderly and for mechanical valve replacement. However, as it stands, Table 28.1 shows the targets!

Table 28.1 INR targets for warfarin therapy

Reason for warfarin therapy	Target INR
AF	2.5
DVT/PE	2.5
Mechanical valve replacement	Dependent on type and location of valve and patient-related risk factors
Recurrence of DVT/PE while on warfarin	3.5

TOP TIPS in Warfarin Dosing

- Don't over-react to individual INRs! Often it is enough to reduce/increase the dose just for 1 or 2 days to allow the INR to get back on target.
- Dose adjustments should be by ±10%. Occasionally you will need to adjust by ±20%, particularly during the early stages of treatment.
- Booster STAT doses should be about 150% of the usual maintenance dose.
- Don't measure the INR too frequently! The effect of a single dose does not start for 12–16 hours and lasts for 4 to 5 days. So unless there are particular concerns, it is pointless measuring the INR more than twice a week during hospital admission.
- The anticoagulant clinic is a good source of advice. Pick up that phone!
- Again, BEWARE in the elderly: they need closer monitoring.

Anticoagulation in the Elderly

The elderly generally:

- need lower doses of warfarin
- have a greater number of other medical conditions and concurrent drug use, which can affect INR stability or alter the risk of bleeding.

Consequently, older folk need to be monitored more carefully.

Reversing the Effects of Warfarin

Before you reach for the vitamin K, stop! Does the patient really need it? Vitamin K certainly will work within 6 hours and will bring the INR into therapeutic range in 24 hours. However, it can also make the patient resistant to warfarin for days, maybe even weeks, especially at doses >2 mg. IV vitamin K is usually only warranted where the patient is bleeding or the INR is very high (Table 28.2).

Table 28.2 Reversing the effects of warfarin

Event	Action
Life-threatening bleeding	Stop warfarin Emergency reversal with 25 U/kg PCC (Beriplex) Give vitamin K 5 mg IV Repeat INR 10 minutes after administration of PCC
Non-major bleeding	Stop warfarin Give vitamin K 1–3 mg IV (consider higher dose if INR >7) Recheck INR following day
INR >8	Stop warfarin Give vitamin K 1–5 mg PO Recheck INR following day
INR 5–8	Stop warfarin for 1–2 days Consider 1 mg vitamin PO in patients at high risk of bleeding (e.g. elderly)

Drug–Drug Interactions

Drugs can affect the INR in warfarinised patients by:

- altering drug binding, or
- altering drug metabolism.

But remember, drugs that affect vitamin K absorption (e.g. those causing or treating malabsorption, or altering bowel flora) will also make a huge difference. It is thus best to treat *any* drug as having the potential to interact with warfarin. However, in practice, the drugs detailed in Table 28.3 tend to cause most of the difficulties seen in clinic.

Drug–Food Interactions

Who said greens were good for you? Patients taking health foods, food supplements and *exceptionally* large quantities of green vegetables (which contain significant quantities of vitamin K) have seen their INR take a skydive. Problem foods include turnips, greens, beetroot, broccoli, cabbage, lettuce and spinach. Healthy portions, however, are fine.

An example: anticoagulant clinic staff were at a loss as to explain why one gentleman's INR was dropping like a stone … until he owned up to being on the cabbage soup diet!

Table 28.3 Drugs that interact with warfarin

Drug	Action
Amiodarone	Increases INR in most patients Onset is slow, but usually develops within 2 weeks. Monitor the patient on a weekly basis for the first 4 weeks of treatment Interaction can persist for many weeks after the amiodarone has been withdrawn.
Antibiotics	Highly unpredictable: broad-spectrum antibiotics often raise INR, but rarely reduce it. In practice, a slight decrease in warfarin dose (e.g. 0.5 mg) for the duration of the course may be advisable
Alcohol	Binge drinking dramatically increases INR Chronic heavy alcohol usage can increase warfarin requirements
Aspirin	Not good news! Analgesic doses of aspirin increase the chance of bleeding, damage the stomach wall and can increase the INR. Triple whammy Low-dose aspirin (75–150 mg) appears to be safer, and in some circumstances is co-prescribed with warfarin
NSAIDs	As for aspirin Avoid if possible. If *absolutely* necessary then ibuprofen/diclofenac are considered the safest options, but use the lowest effective dose and monitor closely

Drug–Disease Interactions

Changes in a patient's clinical condition can interfere with warfarin control. The effect of warfarin is enhanced with:

- liver impairment
- exacerbation of CCF
- renal impairment
- infective episodes
- steatorrhoea.

And reduced with:

- diarrhoea
- vomiting.

Liaising with the Anticoagulant Clinic

The anticoagulant clinic needs a good deal of information to be able to manage a patient properly. Local referral forms are usually available, but the minimum information they need is likely to be:

- diagnosis
- target INR and duration of therapy
- last three INR values and warfarin doses
- other drugs taken
- any risk factors for bleeding.

Most clinics will not accept a patient unless they have all the relevant details. Check what your clinic needs and save yourself some phone calls!

Parenteral Anticoagulation

Robert Shulman

Successful anticoagulation is a fine balance between clotting and bleeding, which can easily go wrong. The good news is that even the thickest clot can be managed with some simple principles!

Low Molecular Weight Heparins

Low molecular weight heparins (LMWHs) are simpler and more convenient to use, and have essentially replaced unfractionated heparin for routine use. There are several agents on the market, but the main ones used are enoxaparin and dalteparin (Fragmin®). See Table 29.1 for treament guidelines.

RED ALERT: LMWHs

DO NOT use treatment-dose LMWHs:

• routinely in the severely obese, based on actual weight: get haematology advice

• in paediatric patients, unless under specialist advice

• at full dose in those with moderate/severe renal impairment (CrCl <30 mL/min).

Table 29.1 Treatment guidelines for LMWHs

Use	
Treatment of DVT/PE	Enoxaparin 1.5 mg/kg SC OD, or 0.75 mg/kg BD *or* Dalteparin 200 units/kg SC OD, max. 18 000 units/day or 100 units/kg SC BD
Treatment of DVT/PE with increased likelihood of bleeding	Dalteparin 100 units/kg SC BD *or* Enoxaparin 0.75 mg/kg BD

(cont.)

Table 29.1 *(cont.)*

Use
Doses above are precise, but your hospital may use standard fixed-dose syringes specific to a weight band. Check local practices
For proven DVT/PE, concomitantly commence warfarin as above. Continue LMWH for at least 4 days, and do not stop until INR has been in the target range for at least 2 days

Monitoring	
FBC before therapy, and repeat every 72 hours thereafter	Checking for heparin-induced thrombocytopenia APTT ratio (APTTr) and anti-Xa levels are not usually required

Reversal	
Severe	Protamine sulfate 40 mg IV Give protamine sulfate IV slowly (5 mg/min), not more than 50 mg at any one time

LMWH might not be fully reversed by protamine. You may need further protamine doses as it is short-acting

Prevention of DVT

All hospitalised patients are at risk of DVT, and this risk should be assessed and minimised for every patient. LMWHs form the bedrock of prevention (Table 29.2).

RED ALERT: Patients Unsuitable for LMWHs

- Platelets <50 × 10⁹/L
- Known bleeding disorder or active bleeding
- LP/epidural within the next 12 h/previous 4 h
- In neurosurgery, DO NOT commence anticoagulation before discussing with the registrar or consultant.

Extra caution is needed in:

- Patients with general risk factors for bleeding (see section entitled 'Risk Factors for Bleeding')
- Renal impairment (CrCl <30 mL/min): use half the normal dose of LMWH (see Table 29.3) or heparin calcium or sodium 5000 units SC BD
- Patients with platelets <75 × 10⁹/L (discuss with haematology team).

Avoid NSAIDs if possible.

Table 29.2 Indications for VTE prophylaxis and therapeutic options

Risk category	Therapy
Medical patients	
All hospitalised medical with reduced mobility adult patients	LMWH OD, e.g. enoxaparin 40 mg SC OD (or dalteparin 5000 units SC OD) until patient mobilises (except for head-injury patients and those in excluded groups above) The role of heparin or warfarin in acute stroke is complex. Discuss with stroke team
Orthopaedic surgery	
• Elective hip (THR) or knee replacement (TKR) • Hip fracture	Post-op, IPC device (if available) while patient fully immobile perioperatively AND continue TEDs LMWH OD 6–8 h post-op, e.g. enoxaparin 40 mg SC OD (or dalteparin 5000 units SC OD) until patient mobilises Nearer discharge, consider changing to rivaroxaban 10 mg PO OD (if clinically appropriate), otherwise continue with enoxaparin/dalteparin. Total duration: THR 35 days/TKR 14 days, assuming back to baseline mobility As above with IPC, TED and LMWH. But continue LMWH (not rivaroxaban) for 28 days
General surgery or trauma	
• Surgical procedure with surgical time >90 minutes, (or 60 minutes for pelvis or lower limb surgery) • Acute surgical admission with inflammatory or intra-abdominal condition • Expected to have significant ↓ in mobility • Have ≥1 risk factors for VTE	LMWH OD, e.g. enoxaparin 40 mg SC OD (or dalteparin 5000 units SC OD) until patient mobilises Consider TEDs

Table 29.3 Dose adjustments for VTE prophylaxis

	Dalteparin dose	Enoxaparin dose
Standard dose	5000 units SC OD	40 mg SC OD
Weight <46 kg/frail elderly/ CrCl 20–30 mL/min	2500 units SC OD	20 mg SC OD
Weight 100–150 kg	5000 units SC BD	40 mg SC BD
Weight 150–200 kg	7500 units SC BD	60 mg SC BD
Weight >200 kg	Seek advice from haematology team	

Risk Factors for VTE

- Age over 60 years
- Obesity (BMI >30 kg/m^2)
- Dehydration
- One or more significant medical co-morbidities (e.g. heart disease; metabolic, endocrine or respiratory pathologies; acute infection; inflammatory conditions)
- Critical care admission
- Active cancer or cancer treatment; haematological malignancy
- Varicose veins with phlebitis
- Personal history or first-degree relative with a history of VTE
- Known thrombophilia or other thrombotic conditions (e.g. haemoglobinopathies, myeloproliferative disease, nephrotic syndrome)
- HRT/oestrogen-containing contraception
- Continuous travel of more than 6 hours approximately 4 weeks before/after surgery
- Pregnancy/less than 6 weeks postpartum.

Risk Factors for Bleeding

- Active bleeding
- Acquired bleeding disorders (such as acute liver or renal failure)
- Concurrent use of anticoagulants (e.g. warfarin with INR >2, DOACs)
- Acute stroke (discuss with neurology)
- Platelets <75 × 10^9/L) – discuss with haematology team
- Uncontrolled systolic hypertension (≥230/120 mmHg)
- Inherited bleeding disorders (e.g. haemophilia and von Willebrand disease)
- Myeloproliferative disorders – discuss with haematology team
- Neurosurgery, spinal or eye surgery
- Other procedures with high risk of bleeding
- Lumbar puncture/epidural/spinal anaesthesia expected within the next 12 h
- Lumbar puncture/epidural/spinal anaesthesia within the previous 4 h.

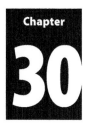

Direct Oral Anticoagulants

Rosalind Byrne and Alison Brown

The direct oral anticoagulants (DOACs) are rivaroxaban, apixaban, edoxaban (factor Xa inhibitors) and dabigatran (direct thrombin inhibitor).

General Rules

- Anticoagulant action DOES NOT need to be routinely monitored, but they remain *high-risk drugs* that can cause or exacerbate bleeding, so
- DO NOT prescribe DOACs with any other anticoagulant (including thromboprophylaxis).
- They have a fast onset and short duration of action therefore *bridging with heparin is not required.*
- They are *NOT suitable for everyone.* We still need to use warfarin sometimes!

DOAC Specifics

- Rivaroxaban must be taken with food for it to be absorbed effectively (particularly at the higher doses).
- Edoxaban and dabigatran require 5 days of low molecular weight heparin (LMWH) before they can be started for acute VTE (see Table 30.1).
- Rivaroxaban and edoxaban are ONCE daily.
- Apixaban and dabigatran are TWICE daily.
- Dabigatran cannot be put in a dossette box.

Who Can Have a DOAC?

All DOACs are NICE approved for:

- Stroke prevention in the context of non-valvular atrial fibrillation with CHA_2DS_2-VASc ≥ 1 (men) or ≥ 2 (women)
- Treatment of VTE (DVT and PE).

Rivaroxaban 10 mg daily and apixaban 2.5 mg BD are licensed for long-term secondary prevention of VTE (following completion of 6 months of treatment) for patients with ongoing risk factors.

Table 30.1 DOAC dosing

DOAC	Standard dose	Dose reduction
Atrial fibrillation (stroke prevention)		
Rivaroxaban	20 mg once daily with food	Rivaroxaban 15 mg once daily with food (CrCl 15–49 mL/min)
Apixaban	5 mg twice daily	2.5 mg twice daily if two or more of (age ≥80 years, weight ≤60 kg and creatinine ≥133 μmol/L) or if CrCl 15–29 mL/min
Edoxaban	60 mg once daily	30 mg once daily where patient is ≤60 kg, CrCl 15–49 mL/min or if on ketoconazole, ciclosporin, dronedarone or erythromycin
Dabigatran	150 mg twice daily	110 mg twice daily for patients aged 80 years or above or on verapamil. Consider dose reduction for patients aged 75–80, with moderate renal impairment (CrCl 30–49 mL/min), those with gastritis, oesophagitis or gastro-oesophageal reflux or who are at an increased risk of bleeding
Treatment of VTE		
Rivaroxaban	15 mg twice daily with food for 21 days and then 20 mg once daily with food thereafter	Dose reduction only considered when risk of bleeding outweighs the risk of recurrent DVT and PE After 6 months – 10 mg daily for secondary VTE prevention (in selected cases)
Apixaban	10 mg twice daily for 7 days, then 5 mg twice daily thereafter	Dose reduction only considered when risk of bleeding outweighs the risk of recurrent DVT and PE After 6 months –2.5 mg twice daily for secondary VTE prevention (in selected cases)
Edoxaban (Requires 5 days LMWH before initiation of edoxaban in acute setting)	60 mg once daily	30 mg once daily where patient is ≤60 kg, CrCl 15–50 mL/min, or if on ketoconazole, ciclosporin, dronedarone or erythromycin
Dabigatran (Requires 5 days LMWH before initiation of dabigatran in acute setting)	150 mg twice daily	110 mg twice daily for patients aged 80 years or above or on verapamil. Consider dose reduction for patients aged 75–80, with moderate renal impairment (CrCl 30–50 mL/min), those with gastritis, oesophagitis or gastro-oesophageal reflux or who are at an increased risk of bleeding

Rivaroxaban, apixaban and dabigatran are licensed for the prevention of VTE post hip and knee replacement.

Rivaroxaban is also licensed, co-administered with aspirin alone or with aspirin plus clopidogrel or ticlopidine, for the prevention of atherothrombotic events in adult patients after an acute coronary syndrome (ACS).

Who Can't Have a DOAC (Will Need Warfarin)

Patients need anticoagulation with warfarin for:

- Mechanical heart valves
- Valvular AF
- Antiphospholipid syndrome
- Acute cancer-associated VTE (LMWH is used currently, but DOACs can be used in selected cases with low bleeding risk, with specialist advice)
- Any reason other than DOACs are licensed for (although sometimes they are used on an off-label basis if low time in range on warfarin or warfarin is completely impractical)

Warfarin should also be used for:

- CrCl* < 15 mL/min (for apixaban, rivaroxaban, edoxaban)
- CrCl* < 30mL/min (for dabigatran)
- Patients on interacting drugs (see Table 30.2)
- Extremes of body weight – there is little evidence for dosing in patients <50 kg and >120 kg. DOACs can be used for licensed indications in selected cases but require monitoring in a specialist anticoagulation clinic.
- Pregnancy or breastfeeding.
  (*creatinine clearance calculated using Cockcroft and Gault equation)

Monitoring

Before initiation, check:

- Renal function (see Table 30.1 for dosing), liver function, FBC, baseline coagulation.

During treatment check:

- Renal function at least every 12 months (6-monthly if CrCl is 30–50 mL/min and/or age >75 years and/or frail, 3-monthly if CrCl is 15–30 mL/min)
- FBC and LFTs at least every 12 months.

In some laboratories, it is possible to measure DOAC plasma levels in patients where there is a concern regarding over- or underdosing (e.g. extremes of body weight, poor renal function, interacting drugs) but this should only be done with specialist advice.

Remember, even though you do not need to monitor INR or APTT for DOACs they will often affect these tests to differing degrees.

Interactions

Obtain specialist advice for managing interactions of other medications with DOACs. Generally, if a significant interaction exists then warfarin is a better option as the INR can be monitored and dosing adjusted to allow for it.

Table 30.2 lists some common interactions and their effects on anticoagulation. This list is not exhaustive. Check all interactions on a case by case basis.

Concurrent Antiplatelets

Most patients do not require antiplatelets as well as anticoagulation. Review all antiplatelets when anticoagulation is started.

However, patients with recent coronary stenting, MI or history of peripheral vascular disease may require concurrent antiplatelets. Discuss with the relevant team before stopping.

Reversal/Haemorrhage

The only DOAC which currently has a specific reversal agent in the UK is dabigatran. Idarucizumab is licensed when the rapid reversal of dabigatran's anticoagulation effect is required. Remember DOACs are short-acting drugs so their effect may often be negligible by the time the patient is seen. Prothrombin complex concentrate (e.g. Octaplex®, Beriplex®) can be used to manage major bleeding in patients on DOACs. Local guidelines should be available. Andexanet alfa, for the reversal of the Xa inhibitors, is currently being reviewed by NICE.

Obtain specialist advice for the management of patients who are bleeding on DOACs.

Perioperative Management

DOACs can generally be stopped 24–48 hours before most operations/procedures without any need for bridging with LMWH. Patients may be prescribed LMWH post procedure at prophylactic or intermediate doses until it is safe to fully anticoagulate with a DOAC. Obtain specialist advice for management of patients on DOACs undergoing operations/procedures.

Discharges/Communication with the Anticoagulation Clinic

There will be a local DOAC prescribing policy. Some areas require hospital initiation and prescribing for a certain period of time and, in some areas, GPs will take on prescribing from initiation.

Table 30.2 Drug interactions with DOACs

DOAC	Concomitant use not recommended* (Reduced anticoagulation effect)	Concomitant use not recommended* (Increased anticoagulation effect)	Cautioned interactions
Rivaroxaban	Rifampicin, phenytoin, carbamazepine, phenobarbital, St John's wort	Ketoconazole, itraconazole, voriconazole, posaconazole HIV protease inhibitors Dronedarone	
Apixaban	Rifampicin, phenytoin, carbamazepine, phenobarbital, St John's wort	Ketoconazole, itraconazole, voriconazole, posaconazole, HIV protease inhibitors Dronedarone	
Dabigatran	Rifampicin, phenytoin, carbamazepine, phenobarbital, St John's wort	Ketoconazole, ciclosporin, itraconazole, dronedarone, tacrolimus, HIV protease inhibitors	Amiodarone, posaconazole, quinidine, ticagrelor *Verapamil – reduce dabigatran dose to 110 mg BD*
Edoxaban	Rifampicin, phenytoin, carbamazepine, phenobarbital, St John's wort	HIV protease inhibitors	Increased effect: *ciclosporin, dronedarone, erythromycin, ketoconazole – reduce dose to 30 mg daily* Drugs which increase gastric emptying and gut motility may reduce absorption of edoxaban

* Combination is occasionally used under anticoagulation advice and with DOAC level monitoring

It is vital that, as a minimum, the following information is communicated to whoever is managing the patient's anticoagulation in the long term:

- Indication for anticoagulation
- DOAC and dose
- Duration of anticoagulation
- Recent bloods and plan for follow-up bloods if necessary.

Advice for Patients

All patients should receive an information leaflet and an alert card (either the card that comes with the drug or a yellow anticoagulation alert card such as the one used for warfarin).

The following counselling points must be covered when starting DOACs:

- What the DOAC is for
- Length of course
- The importance of adherence
- When and how to take the DOAC (particularly if a loading dose, and therefore dose adjustment, is required)
- Rivaroxaban must be taken with food for it to work effectively
- Rivaroxaban can cause dizziness and headache in a small percentage of patients
- Dabigatran can cause indigestion/heart burn
- Patients may bruise more easily and bleed for longer if they injure themselves
- Patients should stop taking the DOAC and attend their nearest A&E if they experience any unexpected and/or uncontrollable bleeding, such as coughing or vomiting blood, blood in the urine or stools, passing black sticky stools, sudden onset of severe headache, nose bleed lasting longer than 10 minutes
- They should attend A&E if they have a fall with an injury to their head or face
- They should take paracetamol for pain relief and avoid taking aspirin, ibuprofen (and any other NSAIDs)
- Avoid contact sports (e.g. rugby, boxing)
- If they become pregnant, they must inform the anticoagulation clinic/GP immediately
- If any procedures/surgery are needed they must contact the anticoagulation clinic/GP for advice.

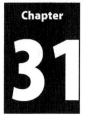

Chapter 31

Practical Prescribing in the Surgical Patient

Mayur Murali

Two issues relate to prescribing for the surgical patient:

- Managing the medication they were taking at home, during the metabolically stressful and potentially starved perioperative period.
- Prescribing drugs required as a consequence of the surgery (e.g. analgesia, antiemetics, thromboprophylaxis, antibiotics and fluids).

Most hospitals have policies and protocols relating to perioperative prescribing. Look them up, and supplement with the following guide.

Enteric Absorption and 'Nil By Mouth'

Patients undergoing a general anaesthetic for elective surgery should not eat solids 6 hours before surgery, to limit the risk of aspiration. However, clear fluids are encouraged until 2 hours before surgery (1 hour in children): this improves gastric motility, thereby reducing aspiration risk and reducing dehydration. Routine medications can be taken with these fluids and, with some notable exceptions, this is generally advised.

If enteral absorption is unlikely, or where reliable absorption is essential, then a switch to parenteral preparations might be needed. Consult your pharmacist: doses may change as the route changes.

Local anaesthetic procedures generally don't require nil by mouth (NBM), but anaesthetists prefer a patient is kept NBM if there is a chance that a general anaesthetic may ensue. Ask!

Routine Drug Modification

Always consider the risk-to-benefit ratio of continuing or discontinuing a medication.

With acknowledgement to Jane Ng, who was the original author of this chapter.

Anticoagulation

(See also Part 6 – Haematology.)

Antiplatelet Agents: Aspirin, Clopidogrel

Aspirin can generally be continued until the day of surgery, particularly in patients at high risk of cardiovascular disease, but may need to be stopped in some specific circumstances (such as intracranial surgery). Clopidogrel should be stopped 7 days prior to most major operations.

For some operations (e.g. carotid endarterectomy), the benefit of continuing the antiplatelet agent outweighs the risk. *Remember: some coronary stents may clot, causing heart attack or death, if dual antiplatelet agents are stopped within a certain timeframe, e.g. the first 30 days for bare metal stents and first 6 months for drug-eluting stents.* The American College of Cardiology and American Heart Association recommend postponing elective surgery for at least 3 months following stent implantation. However, consensus on this is divided, and if in doubt or before emergency surgery, liaise with the cardiology and haematology teams.

Generally, restart antiplatelet agents the next day, unless the patient has an epidural catheter in situ.

Warfarin

Details depend on the indication for warfarin and the operation being performed:

- For AF, previous DVT or PE: stop warfarin 3 to 4 days prior to surgery. Commence standard thromboprophylaxis (see next section) on admission.
- For prosthetic mechanical heart valves: stop warfarin 3 to 4 days prior to surgery. Once the INR is <2, commence a LMWH bridging plan or an unfractionated heparin infusion, if in use at your hospital (to be stopped 2 h prior to surgery).

Warfarin is normally restarted at the normal dose on the evening of surgery or the next day if haemostasis is adequate. If strict control is required, continue the bridging LMWH or heparin infusion postoperatively, simultaneously reload on warfarin and stop the heparin when the INR is therapeutic. However, it may be decided that it is too risky to restart anticoagulation (e.g. following neurosurgery). *If in doubt, discuss with the surgical and haematology teams.*

Direct Oral Anticoagulants: Rivaroxaban, Apixaban, Dabigatran (see also Chapter 30 – DOACs)

Advice for interrupting DOACs is dependent on the indication for their use, their plasma half-life and the patient's co-morbidities, particularly renal function. In general, for minor procedures, DOACs can be continued without interruption, but for major surgical procedures with a high bleeding risk, DOACs should be discontinued for a minimum of 24–48 h (or two half-lives), as a compromise between bleeding risk and thromboembolic complications (this time is increased in renal disease). Bridging therapy is not necessary. Liaise with your local haematologist for further details.

Antidiabetic Agents and Insulin

See Chapter 32 – Diabetes in Surgery.

Steroids

(See also Chapter 43 – Corticosteroids.)

To reduce the risk of postoperative hypoadrenal crisis, steroid replacement is necessary if the patient is currently on steroids or has received a prolonged course of steroids in the preceding 3 months (Table 31.1).

Table 31.1 Steroid replacement therapy

Steroid dose	Type of surgery	
	Minor	Major
Low dose, e.g. prednisolone 5 mg/day	Give usual oral dose prior to surgery, resume oral dose postoperatively	Preoperative: usual oral dose Intraoperative: hydrocortisone 25 mg IV Postoperative: hydrocortisone 25 mg IV 8-hourly for 48 hours, then resume regular oral dose
High dose, e.g. prednisolone 40 mg/day	Give usual oral dose prior to surgery, resume oral dose postoperatively	Preoperative: usual oral dose Intraoperative: hydrocortisone 50 mg IV Postoperative: hydrocortisone 50 mg IV 8-hourly for 72 hours, then resume regular oral dose

Anticonvulsants, Antiparkinsonian Medication and Immunosuppressants

These are usually continued during the perioperative period as the consequences of discontinuation could be serious. Most are available in parenteral or rectal formulations, but bioavailability differs and so expert advice should always be sought before changing the route of administration – ideally *before* the patient goes to theatre!

Drugs Required Following Surgery
Fluids
How much of what?

- Examine the patient (revise the signs of a dry and overloaded patient) and read their chart. Estimate how much fluid they are 'down' from theatre, how 'dry' they are and aim to make this up at an appropriate rate; if hypotensive and compromised, NOW! If slightly dry, over a few hours.
- Now add the 'normal' rate of requirement (25–30 mL/kg/day allows for urinary, faecal and insensible losses).
- Now add 'extra' losses (sweat, diarrhoea, stoma etc.).
- Estimate what they are losing. Salt? Bicarbonate? Water? Potassium?
- Consider deficiencies – are they already low in K$^+$? Do they need blood or clotting products?
- Consider the rate needed and what is safe (e.g. you should be more cautious in a patient with known poor cardiac function).
- Now write up an appropriate regimen.
- Reassess fluid status and remember to monitor urine output.

Fluid requirements should be assessed twice daily, and more frequently in the unwell.

Example

For a routine, 24-hour maintenance fluid regimen in a euvolaemic, well patient, NICE recommends[1]:

- 25–30 mL/kg/day of water
- Approximately 1 mmol/kg/day of potassium, sodium and chloride
- 50–100 g/day of glucose if nil by mouth.

In a 70 kg patient, that equates to 1.7–2.1 litres of water per day with approximately 70 mmol of sodium, potassium and chloride. NICE therefore recommends administering 25–30 mL/kg/day of 0.18% saline in 4% glucose with 27 mmol/L of potassium chloride when fluids are used for maintenance alone.

Be sure to know what your fluid contains before prescribing; composition of the commonly used crystalloids can be found in NICE guidelines.

NB. There is growing evidence that balanced electrolyte solutions – such as Ringer's lactate and Hartmann's – are better fluids than 'normal saline'.

---

[1] NICE Clinical Guideline 174. Intravenous fluid therapy in adults in hospital. 2017. www.nice.org.uk/guidance/cg174/chapter/1-Recommendations#routine-maintenance-2. Accessed August 2019.

Analgesia

(See also Chapter 23 – Analgesia.)

Revise the Analgesic Ladder (see Chapter 23)

Postoperative pain control employs the step-down approach. All patients should be on regular paracetamol (where not contraindicated) and where clinically indicated (and not contraindicated), NSAIDs. In addition, many will need an opiate. *Gradually* wean 'down' the ladder until the patient is off all analgesia (see Table 23.1 for a list of commonly used analgesics).

TOP TIPS for Postoperative Analgesia

- Regular simple analgesia should be the baseline – there is never a place for morphine in the absence of regular paracetamol (PO, PR or now IV). This reduces opioid doses and thus side effects.

- When clinically indicated, a regular NSAID can be added to paracetamol – again sparing opioid doses. Beware in asthmatic patients and renal failure.

- Regular opiate use will usually cause constipation. Consider prescribing a stimulant laxative such as senna. Post surgery, constipation can cause complications such as bowel obstruction, while straining to pass stool isn't the best for an abdominal wound. Lactulose is ineffective for this indication (see Chapter 19 – Constipation in the Adult Patient).

- Codeine is weakly effective in <30% of patients and totally ineffective (due to the genetics of the patient) in 7–10%. It is therefore unreliable! It works by being metabolised to an opioid – so if one is needed, why not use a strong one such as morphine from the start?

- Tramadol often causes severe dysphoria and hallucinations, especially in the elderly. The best advice, then, is to stick to morphine, paracetamol and NSAIDs as your baseline!

Postoperative Nausea and Vomiting

(See also Chapter 20 – Nausea and Vomiting.)

Use a 'step-up' approach: start with one drug, then add a second (and then third) from a different class. For example:

- Ondansetron: PO or IV, 4–8 mg TDS
- Cyclizine: PO, IV or IM, 50 mg TDS
- Prochlorperazine: PO 5–10 mg TDS, IM 12.5 mg (followed in 6 hours by an oral dose), PR 25 mg (followed in 6 hours by an oral dose as above)

TOP TIPS for Postoperative Nausea and Vomiting!

- Domperidone and metoclopramide are not effective in postoperative nausea and vomiting and are inadvisable immediately following GI surgery.
- Give antiemetics regularly rather than intermittently once you have identified the problem. Vomiting is horrid and misery-making and, with an abdominal wound, is very painful and can delay healing. It also upsets fluid and electrolyte balance.
- Always consider *why* they are vomiting. Can you reduce the opioids? Are they obstructed? Do they have an ileus?

Prophylaxis

Thromboprophylaxis

See Chapter 29 – Parenteral Anticoagulation.

Antibiotic Prophylaxis

(See also Chapter 40 – Infections.)

Antibiotic prescribing is usually protocol-driven. Most patients require only one preoperative dose. Therapy continued postoperatively is only of benefit in proven infections.

Patients with cardiac valve lesions/artificial valves will require extra antibiotic cover.

Splenectomy Prophylaxis

1. Prescribe (2 weeks prior to elective splenectomy or 2 weeks after emergency splenectomy):
   a. pneumococcal vaccine 0.5 mL IM
   b. haemophilus influenza B vaccine 0.5 mL IM
   c. meningococcal conjugated C vaccine 0.5 mL IM
2. Prescribe lifelong penicillin V PO 250–500 mg BD (or erythromycin 250–500 mg BD if penicillin-allergic)
3. Give a splenectomy card to take away.

High-Output Stomas

(See also Chapter 18 – Practical Prescribing in Gastroenterology.)

Jejunostomies usually require specialist input. They produce large volumes of stomal output, high in sodium and greater after eating and drinking. Treatment options include:

- dietetics input for low-residue, high-salt diet
- high-dose loperamide 4–8 mg QDS and/or codeine 60–120 mg QDS

- addition of a proton pump inhibitor or H_2 antagonist
- oral fluid restriction and refer to specialist team for advice on whether to give hypertonic salt solutions PO
- replace sodium, magnesium and calcium as required IV
- octreotide as a last resort (only after all the above measures have failed) – reduces stomal output.

Ileostomies: if no identifiable cause, use loperamide 2–4 mg PO before meals or codeine 60 mg PO before meals. Involve dietetics and stoma therapy.

Colostomies: rule out causes other than surgery, such as antibiotics, obstruction and overflow. Use loperamide with caution. Get advice from stoma therapy and dietetics.

Chapter 32

Diabetes in Surgery

Jessal Mitul Palan

General Management

Patients with an HbA1c >8.5% (69 mmol/mol) should be reviewed by the local diabetes team before surgery, ideally in an outpatient setting, in order to optimise diabetes management. If surgery is necessary before glycaemic targets can be achieved, inpatient diabetes input should be sought preoperatively. Adverse outcomes associated with poor preoperative diabetes management include higher morbidity and mortality (in particular, cardiovascular), higher risk of diabetic ketoacidosis and hypoglycaemia, prolonged inpatient stay, and higher surgical and systemic complications, e.g. poor wound healing.

TOP TIPS for Perioperative Diabetic Patients

- Highlight patients with diabetes to the anaesthetist, as they should take precedence on the operative list.
- Consider admitting patients with hyperglycaemia/HbA1c >7.5% the night prior to surgery in order to optimise fasting glycaemia.
- Monitor capillary blood glucose (CBG) every 2 hours pre- and postoperatively, with an aim to keep this within an acceptable range (6–12 mmol/L).[1] Local guidelines may vary, so local diabetes input should be sought to lower the likelihood of adverse outcomes.
- Ensure that all patients with type 1 diabetes and patients with type 2 diabetes taking sulfonylureas, DPP-4 inhibitors and insulin have Glucogel®, glucagon and NovoRapid® prescribed to help treat hypoglycaemia (CBG <4 mmol/L) swiftly if required. NovoRapid is likely to act quicker than Actrapid®, although it is slightly more expensive to use.

---

[1] JBDS Management of adults with diabetes undergoing surgery and elective procedures: improving standards. www.diabetes.org.uk/professionals/position-statements-reports/specialist-care-for-children-and-adults-and-complications/management-of-adults-with-diabetes-undergoing-surgery-and-elective-procedures-improving-standards. Accessed February 2019.

Perioperative Management
Type 1 (Table 32.1)

Table 32.1 Perioperative management of type 1 diabetes

Type of insulin	Day before surgery	Day of surgery	Restarting after surgery
Long-acting, e.g. glargine (Lantus, Abasaglar), degludec (Tresiba), detemir (Levemir)	Consider reducing by 20%	Continue long-acting analogue at reduced dose as per day before surgery DO NOT STOP LONG-ACTING ANALOGUE FOR ANY REASON	Return back to usual dose if eating and drinking and no AKI
Short-acting, e.g. NovoRapid, Actrapid, Humulin S, Humalog	Usual dose	Omit on day of surgery	Restart at usual dose if eating and drinking and no AKI. If on variable-rate insulin infusion (VRII), see advice below on discontinuing VRII postoperatively
Pump	Inform diabetes team of admission – will need review prior to surgery	Continue basal pump rate only	Restart boluses with meals as per local diabetes team advice

It is important to ensure the patient is not hyperglycaemic (or hypoglycaemic) before surgery on the day of the procedure.

RED ALERT: Perioperative Hyperglycaemia

Hyperglycaemia may be present due to diabetic ketoacidosis, which requires the following criteria to be met:

- Known history of diabetes OR capillary blood glucose >11 mmol/L
- pH <7.3 or bicarbonate <15 on blood gas measurement (venous or arterial)
- Ketonaemia ≥3 mmol/L OR 2+ on urine dipstick.

If the CBG is >15 mmol/L – check the bedside blood/urine ketones. Blood ketones are more accurate to measure:

- If blood ketones >3 or urinary ketones 2+ or more, surgery should not proceed. Contact the diabetes team and the patient should be treated as per local diabetic ketoacidosis (DKA) guidelines with a fixed-rate insulin infusion to suppress ketogenesis (see Chapter 9 – Diabetic Ketoacidosis).
- If blood ketones <2 or urine ketones 1+:
  - If the patient has type 1 diabetes, give patient's usual short-acting insulin, e.g. NovoRapid. Some patients will be aware of how many units of insulin they usually take to correct blood sugar levels and will have their own ratio of how many mmol/L they would expect their glucose to drop with 1 unit of insulin. If unknown, assume each unit of insulin will reduce blood glucose by approximately 3 mmol/L. Recheck CBG in 1 hour. If surgery is an emergency or imminent, commence a VRII as per local guidelines.
  - If patient has type 2 diabetes, give 0.1 units/kg short-acting insulin, e.g. NovoRapid, and recheck CBG in 1 hour. If surgery is an emergency or imminent, commence a VRII as per local guidelines.

If a variable-rate insulin infusion (VRII) is commenced (see Chapter 35 – Intravenous Insulin Infusions):

- Use 5% glucose and 0.45% saline with 0.15/0.3% potassium chloride alongside this at a rate to meet fluid requirements for the patient as set out by the surgical team.
- Alternatively, 4% glucose and 0.18% saline with 0.15/0.3% potassium chloride can be used.
- DO NOT use a regimen consisting of alternating bags of glucose and saline.
- Close monitoring of venous blood gas sodium is advised while on VRII and fluids.

Type 2

Diet-Controlled Diabetes

Managing glycaemia for patients with diet-controlled diabetes rarely requires any intervention – monitor the CBGs.

Oral Medication (Table 32.2)

Table 32.2 Perioperative management of oral medication for type 2 diabetes

Medication	Day before surgery	Day of surgery	Restarting after surgery
Metformin	Continue	Day case/fast for single meal – continue Longer procedure/ eGFR <60 mL/ min/1.73 m²/ contrast use perioperatively – stop on morning of surgery/ when fasting commenced	Restart the day after surgery if eating and drinking and eGFR >60 mL/ min/1.73 m². If AKI, hold. Metformin dose should be reduced if eGFR 30–50 mL/ min/1.73 m² to a maximum of 500 mg twice a day (BD), and stopped altogether if the eGFR <30 mL/ min/1.73m²
Sulfonylureas (e.g. gliclazide, glibenclamide, glipizide, glimepiride)	Continue	Omit on day of surgery	Restart the day after surgery if eating and drinking, and no AKI (can restart in evening if short procedure in the morning)
SGLT2 inhibitors (e.g. empagliflozin, dapagliflozin, canagliflozin)	Continue	Omit 24 h before surgery	Restart the day after surgery (NB hold if AKI)
DPP-4 inhibitors (e.g. sitagliptin, linagliptin, alogliptin)	Continue	Continue	Continue (NB may require dose reduction if AKI)
Pioglitazone	Continue	Continue	Continue
GLP-1 agonists (e.g. exenatide, liraglutide, dulaglutide)	Continue	Continue	Continue

Insulin-Requiring (Table 32.3)

If CBG > 15 mmol/L, follow advice as above for type 1 diabetes.

Table 32.3 Perioperative management of insulin for type 2 diabetes

Type of insulin	Day before surgery	Day of surgery	Restarting after surgery
Mixed, e.g. Humalog Mix25/Mix50, Humulin M3, NovoMix 30, Insuman Comb	Usual dose	Half dose with omitted meals on day of surgery. If switched to using VRII, likely to require basal insulin – contact your local diabetes input for advice	Usual dose if eating and drinking and no AKI
Basal-bolus regimen (long- and short-acting analogues)	Consider reducing both by 20%	As above for type 1 diabetes – continue long-acting analogue (e.g. glargine (Lantus, Abasaglar), degludec (Tresiba), detemir (Levemir)) and omit short-acting analogue (e.g. NovoRapid, Actrapid, Humulin S, Humalog). DO NOT STOP LONG-ACTING ANALOGUE FOR ANY REASON	Restart at usual dose if eating and drinking and no AKI

Postoperative Management

Postoperative glucose levels may well be erratic – adjustments will likely be required as the patient resumes a normal diet. Aim to keep CBGs at 6–12 mmol/L.

RED ALERT: Postoperative Hyperglycaemia

Hyperglycaemia may be present due to diabetic ketoacidosis (see previous box for criteria).

If the CBG is >15 mmol/L – check bedside blood/urine ketones:

- If blood ketones >3 or urinary ketones 2+ or more, contact the diabetes team and the patient should be treated as per local DKA guidelines with fixed-rate insulin to suppress ketogenesis (see Chapter 9 – Diabetic Ketoacidosis).
- If blood ketones <2 or urine ketones 1+:
  - If the patient has type 1 diabetes, give patient's usual short-acting insulin, e.g. NovoRapid. Some patients will be aware of how many units

of insulin they usually take to correct blood sugar levels and will have their own ratio of how many mmol/L they would expect their glucose to drop with 1 unit of insulin. If unknown, assume each unit of insulin will reduce blood glucose by approximately 3 mmol/L. Recheck CBG in 1 hour. Repeat insulin dose in 2 hours if CBG >15 mmol/L. If more than two subcutaneous insulin doses do not bring glycaemia into range (6–12 mmol/L), consider starting a VRII.

· If the patient has type 2 diabetes, give 0.1 units/kg short-acting insulin, e.g. NovoRapid, and recheck CBG in 1 hour. Repeat insulin dose in 2 hours if CBG > 15 mmol/L (consider a higher dose if initial dose did not lead to a fall in blood glucose). If more than two subcutaneous insulin doses do not bring glycaemia into range (6–12 mmol/L), consider starting a VRII.

Diabetes team input should be requested if continued use of VRII required for a prolonged period postoperatively.

Hypos

Patients with diet-controlled diabetes are unlikely to fall into this group, but if symptomatic (e.g. sweating, shaking, confusion), they and all other patients with diabetes should be managed as in Chapter 11 – Hypoglycaemia.

Discontinuing VRII (if Eating and Drinking and No Nausea/Vomiting)

Type 2 Diabetes on Oral Medication Only

• Can stop at any time and restart oral medication as per advice above. Monitor CBG hourly until euglycaemic for two readings (6–12 mmol/L).

Type 2 Diabetes on Mixed Insulin

• Only stop with breakfast/dinner and administer usual subcutaneous mixed insulin with meal. Continue VRII for 1 hour after meal and administered subcutaneous insulin, then stop. Monitor CBG hourly until euglycaemic for two readings (6–12 mmol/L). If patient remains hyperglycaemic, they may need a correction dose of short-acting insulin – contact your local diabetes team for advice.

Type 2 Diabetes on Basal-Bolus Regimen/Type 1 Diabetes

• Administer usual subcutaneous bolus (short-acting) insulin with meal. Continue VRII for 1 hour after meal and administered subcutaneous insulin, then stop. Monitor CBG hourly until euglycaemic for two readings (6–12 mmol/L). If patient remains hyperglycaemic, they may need correction dose of short-acting insulin – if the patient is aware of how many units of insulin they usually take to correct blood sugar levels, follow this pattern. Contact your local diabetes team for advice otherwise.

Insulin Pump

- Contact your local diabetes team in advance. Patient should administer their usual dose of bolus insulin from the pump with each meal. Continue VRII for 1 hour after meal and insulin bolus, then stop. Monitor CBG hourly until euglycaemic for two readings. If patient remains hyperglycaemic, they may need correction dose of bolus pump insulin – if the patient is aware of how many units of insulin they usually take to correct blood sugar levels, follow this pattern. Occasionally, hyperglycaemia may be due to problems with the pump cannula and this may need to be resited. If unsure regarding bolus doses/resiting the pump cannula, contact your local diabetes team.

Chapter 33

Bowel Preparation
Mayur Murali

Oral bowel preparation, once commonly prescribed before elective colorectal surgery to reduce the likelihood of anastomotic leak, is now not required for most procedures: indeed, its use has been associated with harm (hypovolaemia, electrolyte imbalance and nephropathy). Therefore, *be cautious*; make sure you have weighed both risk and benefit of prescribing it, and of the surgical procedure itself. Procedures that may require bowel preparation include surgery to the small or large bowel (and may also include gynaecological or urological procedures), colonoscopy or some radiological investigations. The following advice is based on 2012 guidelines released by the British Society of Gastroenterology.[1]

Absolute contraindications to the use of oral bowel preparation include:

- Ileus, GI obstruction or perforation
- Severe acute inflammatory bowel disease (IBD) or toxic megacolon
- Risk of aspiration
- Allergy to any of the ingredients
- Ileostomy.

Relative contraindications include:

- Chronic kidney disease, haemodialysis or peritoneal dialysis
- Renal transplant
- Congestive cardiac failure
- Liver cirrhosis and/or ascites
- Medications including ACE inhibitors, ARBs, diuretics, NSAIDs and medications that induce the syndrome of inappropriate antidiuretic hormone secretion (SIADH)
- Frail elderly patients.

With acknowledgement to Olivia Hanmeer, who was the original author of this chapter.
[1] A. Connor, D. Tolan, S. Hughes, et al. Consensus guidelines for the safe prescription and administration of oral bowel cleansing agents. *Gut* 2012; 61(11): 1525–32.

The type of bowel preparation is dependent upon the time and type of treatment or investigation. Remember **SICKLy** – CHECK with local preferences before prescribing, as ineffective treatments will result in delays and missed theatre slots. In patients at risk of developing renal failure (e.g. diabetic, hypertensive or patients with structural renal tract disease), make sure a recent (within 3 months) measure of kidney function is available.

General Advice

- Omit solids for at least 6 hours prior to the operation.
- Allow clear fluids only during this time.
- Hypovolaemia must be corrected before, and prevented during, administration of oral bowel preparation agents. Pay particular attention to those who may not be able to maintain adequate oral fluid intake at home.
- Regular oral medications should not be taken 1 h before or after administration of bowel preparation agents due to the risk of malabsorption.
- Those on the oral contraceptive pill should be advised to use alternative precautions for the week following administration.
- Liaise with the diabetic team for patients receiving treatment with insulin.

Preparations on offer are shown in Table 33.1.

Seek advice from your local pharmacist on the most appropriate regimen for your patients.

Table 33.1 Bowel preparation

Laxative	Typical dose	Additional information
Klean-Prep® (polyethylene glycol)	Four sachets in 4 L within 4–6 hours; or Two sachets in the evening before procedure and a further two on the morning of the examination	Until 4 L drunk or bowel motions become clear and watery Less likely to cause hypovolaemia
Citramag® (magnesium carbonate and citric acid)	One sachet at 8 am the day before the procedure then one sachet 6–8 hours later	For elderly patients, use half of the stated dose Avoid in patients at risk of hypovolaemia
Fleet® Phospho-soda (sodium phosphate mixture)	First dose – 45 mL diluted with half a glass of cold water. Second dose – 30 mL diluted with half a glass of cold water Both doses followed by a glass of cold water Morning procedure: first dose at 7 am the day before, second dose at 7 am on the day of the procedure. Afternoon procedure: first dose at 12 pm on the day before the procedure and second dose at 12 pm on the day of the procedure	Use discouraged in patients with: • CKD • Congestive cardiac failure • Liver cirrhosis • Hypertension • Electrolyte disturbance
Picolax® (sodium picosulfate and magnesium citrate)	One sachet at 8 am the day before the procedure then one sachet 6–8 hours later	Heat is generated on reconstitution and will work within 3 hours of the first dose Avoid in patients at risk of hypovolaemia

Chapter 34

Treating Diabetes

Lloyd E. Kwanten and
Miriam Conway

Tables 34.1 and 34.2 will familiarise you with the more common insulin preparations and oral hypoglycaemics.

Insulin Preparations

Preparations differ in their pharmacokinetics. Note that the action profiles can be affected by the dose, injection site and technique, exercise and temperature.

Oral Diabetes Agents

Oral diabetes agents are prescribed in Type 2 diabetes when the patient fails to respond adequately to at least 3 months' restriction of energy and carbohydrate intake and an increase in physical activity. They should be used to augment the effect of diet and exercise, and not to replace them.

Specialist advice should be sought when commencing a newly diagnosed diabetic patient on medication, or if withholding medications (e.g nil by mouth or prior to surgery).

With acknowledgement to Preet Panesar, who was the original author of this chapter.

Table 34.1 Insulin preparations

Insulin type	Onset	Peak	Duration
Rapid acting			
Humalog® (insulin lispro) NovoRapid® (insulin aspart)	Within 15 min	0.5–1 hour	2–5 hours
Short acting			
Human Actrapid® Humulin S®	30 min	1–3 hours	6–8 hours
Intermediate acting			
Human Insulatard® Humulin I®	2 hours	4–12 hours	Up to 24 hours (considerable patient variation)
Long acting			
Human Monotard® Human Ultratard®	2–4 hours	6–20 hours	Up to 36 hours
Long-acting analogues			
Lantus® (insulin glargine) Detemir® (insulin levemir)	1 hour	Flat	24 hours
Mixed insulins (biphasic)			
NovoMix 30® Humalog Mix® 25, 50 Human Mixtard® 10, 20, 30, 40, 50 Humulin M3®	Up to 2 hours	4–12 hours	Up to 24 hours

Table 34.2 Oral diabetes agents

	Indications	Action	Side effects[a]	Advantages	Contraindications	Timing	Example
Biguanides	Typically (though not exclusively) obese patients First line Can be used for gestational diabetes in pregnancy	↑insulin sensitivity	Nausea, abdominal pain, diarrhoea	Does not cause hypos, reduces requirement of other diabetes agents/higher insulin doses	eGFR 30–50 reduce dose eGFR <30 contraindicated Liver derangement/ failure Raised lactate/lactic acidosis Ketoacidosis Care with contrast media	Take on a full stomach or after meals to reduce risk of GI side effects Consider MR if GI tolerability prevents patient continuing	Metformin
Sulfonylureas	Typically non-obese, first or second line Unable to tolerate metformin Steroid-induced diabetes	Beta cell insulin secretagogue	Weight gain, hypo risk	Reduces insulin requirement Steroid-induced diabetes	Renal impairment Ketoacidosis Avoid long-acting preparations in the elderly G6PD deficiency Pregnancy/breastfeeding	15–30 minutes before food	Gliclazide, glibenclamide, glipizide, glimepiride, tolbutamide
Acarbose	Second or third line	↓intestinal absorption	Abdominal pain, flatulence, diarrhoea	Does not cause hypos but can enhance risk in patients using secretagogues/insulin	Hepatic impairment eGFR <25 Pregnancy/breastfeeding IBD or obstruction	Just before food or with first mouthful of food	Acarbose

(cont.)

Table 34.2 (cont.)

	Indications	Action	Side effects[a]	Advantages	Contraindications	Timing	Example
Thiazolidine-diones (glitazones)	Second or third line Unable to tolerate metformin In combination either with metformin or a sulfonylurea	↓Insulin resistance	Weight gain, peripheral and macular oedema, liver impairment, increased LDL-cholesterol (only with rosiglitazone), bladder cancer, bone fractures	Increases HDL-C Reduces triglycerides	Liver impairment Heart failure Pregnancy/breastfeeding Not licensed for use with insulin	Just before food	Pioglitazone, rosiglitazone
Prandial glucose regulators (meglitinides)	Second or third line Unable to tolerate metformin	↑Insulin release	Hypos, weight gain, abdominal pain, diarrhoea, nausea	Useful in those with chaotic lifestyles	Ketoacidosis Moderate/severe liver impairment Pregnancy/breastfeeding Caution in renal impairment	Within 30 minutes before meals	Repaglinide, nateglinide
DPP-4 inhibitors	Second or third line	↓Glucagon release ↑Insulin release	Nausea and diarrhoea, peripheral oedema, headache, dizziness, hypoglycaemia		Ketoacidosis Acute pancreatitis Pregnancy/breastfeeding	Reduce dose if eGFR reduced (except linagliptin)	Sitagliptin, vildagliptin, saxagliptin, linagliptin
SGLT2 inhibitors	Second or third line	↑Renal glucose excretion	GU infections, polyuria, volume depletion, increased risk of AKI, increased risk of DKA, hypos with secretagogues/insulin	Weight loss Blood pressure reduction Reduction in cardiovascular events	DKA/ketosis-prone	Stop 24–48 hours prior to surgery	Dapagliflozin, empagliflozin

[a] See BNF for complete list.

Chapter 35

Intravenous Insulin Infusions
Lloyd E. Kwanten

Control of glucose levels in diabetics is difficult during inter-current illness or a perioperative period. It requires an appreciation of changes, such as counter-regulatory hormones, unpredictable eating (e.g. illness, NBM, changing meal times), changing IV glucose rates, lack of exercise, unusual timing of insulin injections and use of medications such as glucocorticoids and catecholamines. Tight control is important: it improves outcomes in critically ill hospitalised patients and reduces infection rates.

A variety of different methods have emerged to administer continuous IV insulin. These regimes can be fixed-rate insulin infusions (FRII) such as that used in DKA, or variable-rate insulin infusions (VRII), also known as a 'sliding scale'. VRII are commonly used for patients who are 'nil-by-mouth', though they have been criticised for 'chasing' blood glucose levels, which may lead to erratic changes in blood glucose levels. When commencing a VRII, continue the patient's usual basal SC insulin while stopping rapid-acting or mixed insulins. An example of a VRII is given below, but you should *find and use your local hospital guidelines*.

VRII example:

- Insulin is given via a syringe driver: 50 units of soluble insulin (normally Actrapid) made up to 50 mL NaCl 0.9% (i.e. 1 IU/mL).
- The insulin infusion is started at a rate depending on initial CBG (see Table 35.1). If the patient has previously been on insulin then divide the dose of insulin by 24 and start at this rate (e.g. 48 units in 24 hours = start infusion at 2 IU/h).
- The insulin infusion rate is changed according to a predefined scale which is dependent on blood glucose levels (see Table 35.1).
- Some hospitals have two or three different regimens. Patients will normally start on regimen 2, unless they have insulin resistance or still have uncontrolled blood glucose levels (based on JBDS (2014) recommendations).[1]

With acknowledgement to Preet Panesar, who was the original author of this chapter.
[1] Joint British Diabetes Societies for inpatient care (JBDS-IP). The use of variable rate intravenous insulin infusion (VRIII) in medical inpatients. 2014. www.diabetologists-abcd.org.uk/JBDS/JBDS_IP_VRIII.pdf. Accessed August 2019.

Table 35.1 Variable-rate insulin infusion

Blood glucose level (mmol/L)	Insulin infusion rate (units/hour)		
	Regimen 1[a]	Regimen 2[b]	Regimen 3[c]
4.1–8	0.5	1	2
8.1–12	1	2	4
12.1–16	2	4	6
16.1–20	3	5	7
20.1–24	4	6	8
>24.1	Medical review		

[a] Reduced rate in insulin-sensitive patients, e.g. <24 U/day
[b] First choice in most patients
[c] Insulin-resistant patients, e.g. <100 U/day

- Blood glucose levels should be checked hourly. Aim for blood glucose levels of 6–10 mmol/L (though 4–12 mmol/L is acceptable).
- Test for capillary blood ketones in Type 1 diabetics with two CBG readings >12 mmol/L, or in any diabetic patient presenting with acute illness.
- Treat hypoglycaemia, and once CBG >4 mmol/L restart VRII within 20 minutes to prevent ketosis, as the half-life of intravenous insulin is very short.
- Regular monitoring of electrolytes is required.
- Concurrent fluids should be administered to avoid hypoglycaemia and maintain fluid and electrolyte balance. Balanced electrolyte solutions are recommended, such as:
  - 0.45% NaCl with 5% glucose and 0.15%/0.30% KCl (20 mmol/40 mmol) OR
  - 5% glucose with 20 mmol/40 mmol KCl OR
  - 0.18% NaCl with 4% glucose and 0.15%/0.30% KCl (20 mmol/40 mmol).

Once the rate of infusion has been decided, the rate should not be altered unless there are concerns about fluid overload. Fluids containing 0.9% NaCl should be avoided unless clinically indicated (e.g. the patient is vomiting, pyrexial or dehydrated).

Chapter

Calculations for the Prescriber

Updated by Gemma Wareing

Individuals still need to perform drug calculations 'de novo', or for the 'common sense check' of those done by electronic systems. This is true for every ward, but more so for high-risk specialties including paediatrics, emergency medicine, anaesthetics and ICU. Here are some hints and tips.

1. Be Clear About Your Units

TOP TIPS

- 1 kilogram (kg)   =   1000 grams (g)
- 1 gram (g)   =   1000 milligrams (mg)
- 1 milligram (mg)   =   1000 micrograms (μg or mcg)
- 1 microgram (μg)   =   1000 nanograms (ng)
- 1 litre (L)   =   1000 millilitres (mL)

Do the Maths in Two Directions, and Make Sure it Works

For example, your 85-year-old patient with metastatic bowel cancer is now for palliative care. He has been asking for a total of 60 mg of 'PRN' morphine a day, and the palliative care nurse is recommending a SC morphine infusion.

a. You need to give 60 mg morphine in 24 hours.

b. Morphine comes in various concentrations – one is 30 mg in 1 mL. Therefore, you need two vials of the drug, totalling 2 mL.

c. SC pumps come in various sizes – one is a 30 mL pump. Therefore, you need to prescribe 2 mL of drug made up to a total of 30 mL with water.

d. Run this pump over 24 hours, i.e. the pump will run at a rate of 1.25 mL/hour.

With acknowledgement to Simon Keady, who was the original author of this chapter.

Now, work this backwards:

a. 1.25 mL contains 2.5 mg of drug.

b. 2.5 mg of drug/hour equates to 60 mg of drug in 24 hours.

You've done it right!

Do a Rough Maths Check in Your Head

If you need 12 mg for a dose and the ampoules come as 100 mg in 5 mL, you know this is 10 mg in 0.5 mL and therefore 20 mg in 1 mL. Therefore, 12 mg should fall somewhere in between but closer to the 10 mg volume than 20 mg volume… answer 0.6 mL.

2. Do a 'Common Sense' Check

'How many vials of a drug am I asking a nurse to reconstitute? *THAT* many? Am I really going to give that three-year-old a dose I would normally give to an adult? Is that patient really going to need a whole bottle of medicine four times a day?'

3. Always, Always, ALWAYS Get Someone to Double-Check With You

When you are most tired, you are most confident – and also most likely to make an error.

Percentages and Ratios

Percentages can be very confusing! Two key facts help:

Fact 1

A percentage value is a weight or a volume in 100 mL, e.g.:

- 0.9% sodium chloride is 0.9 g per 100 mL
- 5% dextrose is 5 g per 100 mL.

So 5% dextrose won't help to treat or prevent hypoglycaemia very well: you need more sugar (e.g. 10% or 50% dextrose, i.e. 10 g per 100 mL or 50 g per 100 mL).

Fact 2

Diluting will always give you a lower percentage. So for that patient needing an epidural, starting with 25 mL bupivacaine (0.25%), diluting down to 50 mL with 0.9% sodium chloride will double the volume, and halve the final concentration to 0.125%.

Ratios can be just as tricky.

Key Fact

The weight is always in grams and the volume in millilitres.

For instance, adrenaline is commonly available in two strengths:

- adrenaline 1 in 10 000 = 1 g in 10 000 ml = 0.1 mg/mL
- adrenaline 1 in 1000 = 1 g in 1000 ml = 1 mg/mL

In the periarrest situation, you might want to give 'a bit' of adrenaline. If there's not enough time to draw the exact concentration you want, grab the 1 in 1000 adrenaline from the crash trolley and dilute it, e.g. take out 10 mL from a 100 mL bag of 0.9% sodium chloride and replace it with the 10 mL minijet 1 in 1000 adrenaline from the crash trolley. Give it a shake. You now have adrenaline at 0.01 mg (10 micrograms) in 1 mL.

Infusion Administration

Other infusions are delivered through medical devices (usually a volumetric pump or syringe driver), and these deliver a volume as mL per hour. The majority of these devices require syringes to be made to a final volume of 50 mL.

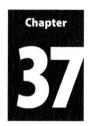

Therapeutic Drug Monitoring

Nishma Gadher

Therapeutic drug monitoring (or TDM) is aimed at monitoring drug levels in the blood to ensure that they are at a therapeutic (and not a toxic) level, thus increasing efficacy of the drug and improving patient outcome. Not all medications require TDM.

Those which do have a recognised desired serum concentration range that will produce its optimal effect with minimal toxicity.

Why do We Take Levels?

- Is the patient experiencing adverse effects of the drug?
- Are you trying to achieve a therapeutic target to ensure efficacy, e.g. antiepileptics?
- Is there a drug interaction to consider?
- Has there been a decline in renal or hepatic function?

The drugs you are most likely to encounter that require TDM are:

- Gentamicin
- Phenytoin
- Digoxin
- Theophylline/aminophylline
- Lithium
- Amikacin
- Vancomycin.

When do We Take Levels?

A level taken at random is no help to anyone. It takes about four to five half-lives for a regularly administered drug to accumulate in the blood, at which point the

---

With acknowledgement to Nicola Mayne, who wrote the original chapter.

drug is said to be in steady state. Once the drug has reached steady state, you either take a:

- *Trough level*: sample immediately before the dose is due, when the drug concentration is at its lowest

  OR

- *Peak level*: timing depends on the half-life of a drug – the longer the half-life, the longer you must wait before the drug concentration is at its highest.

Remember! Label the sample with the *time of sampling* and the *time of dosing*. Without it, the lab staff cannot help you to interpret the result.

RED ALERT: For Obese Patients, Use Corrected Body Weight

Ideal body weight (IBW) kg:

   IBW (male) = 50 kg in weight + (2.3 × every inch over 5 ft in height)
   IBW (female) = 45 kg in weight + (2.3 × every inch over 5 ft in height)

Corrected body weight (CBW):

   CBW (kg) = IBW + (0.4 × (Actual Body Weight − IBW))

Use if patient is obese, defined as >20% over IBW.

What do the Levels Mean?

This is not always simple. When in doubt, get help!

If levels are HIGH, consider:

- Was the dose too high?
- Were the levels taken at the correct time?
- Is there a possible drug interaction?

If levels are LOW, consider:

- Is the dosing too low for the patient?
- Is there a compliance issue?

Common Examples

Gentamicin

Be aware of the two methods of gentamicin dosing (Table 37.1).

Table 37.1 TDM for gentamicin

Multiple daily dosing

1–1.5 mg/kg IV with frequency depending on estimated creatinine clearance (CrCl; see Chapter 2 – Prescribing in Renal Disease)

In obesity use corrected body weight

If CrCl:

- \>70 mL/min, 8-hourly
- 30–70 mL/min, 12-hourly
- <30 mL discuss with microbiology or pharmacy

Other dosing commonly used: 1 mg/kg IV BD for endocarditis

When?	Take first pre and post levels around third or fourth dose	
	If renal impairment, take around second dose	
	Pre (trough) = immediately before next dose	
	Post (peak) = 1 hour after dose	
	Check levels after every dose change and repeat twice weekly unless renal impairment, when they should be checked daily or as advised	
Meaning?	Pre: <2 mg/L	Post: 5–10 mg/L
	Endocarditis:	
	Pre: <1 mg/L	Post: 3–5 mg/L
Action?	If the trough level is >2 mg/mL, withhold the next doses until the level falls <2 mg/mL	
	Adjust the dosage interval rather than the actual dose	

(cont.)

Table 37.1 (cont.)

Once-daily dosing

5 or 7 mg/kg IV
If obese, use corrected body weight

When?	5 mg/kg	Take trough level 30 minutes prior to next dose
	7 mg/kg	Levels any time between 6 and 14 hours postdose after the first dose given
Meaning?	5 mg/kg	Trough level should be <1 mg/L
	7 mg/kg	Refer to the Hartford nomogram (Figure 37.1)

Action?	5 mg/kg	Calculated CrCl	Advised Initial Dosing Interval	Trough level		
				<1 mg/L	1 to 2 mg/L	2 to 3 mg/L
		>60 mL/min	24 hours	Continue	Change to 36-hourly	Seek advice
		40–59 mL/min	36 hours	Continue	Seek advice	Seek advice
	7 mg/kg	If the levels are high, increase the interval between doses as per the Hartford nomogram				

NOTE: Contraindications to using 7 mg/kg/day regimen:

- Age > 70 years
- CrCl < 20 mL/min
- Endocarditis
- Pregnancy
- Patients with ascites, severe liver disease and jaundice
- Prophylaxis
- Major burns
- Cystic fibrosis

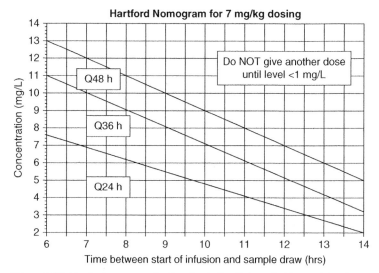

Figure 37.1 Hartford nomogram for 7 mg/kg dosing. (Adapted with permission from Nicolau D, Freeman C, Beliveau P, et al. Experience with a once-daily aminoglycoside program administered to 2,184 adult patients. *Antimicrobial Agents and Chemotherapy* 1995, 39(3): 650–655.)

Pay attention to older patients whose kidneys have seen better days and who are most likely to require a dose adjustment. On the flip side, the higher the peak, the faster the kill of the bacteria, so ad hoc dose reductions are not the answer.

Digoxin

Table 37.2 TDM for digoxin

Loading dose	Urgent: 0.5–1 mg IV over 2 hours
Maintenance dose	62.5–250 micrograms PO OD Lower dose in the elderly or the renally impaired
Why?	Avoid toxicity Investigate treatment failure
When?	Take levels one week after starting treatment Sample 6 hours post dose Not necessary in all patients starting therapy Advisable in the elderly and the renally impaired

(cont.)

Table 37.2 *(cont.)*

Meaning?	Recommended therapeutic range:
	• 0.5–1.5 mg/L target in heart failure
	• 1.5–2 mg/L target in arrhythmias
	>3 mg/L is usually associated with signs of toxicity, which can include lethargy, confusion, GI symptoms and cardiac arrhythmias
	Toxicity possible at levels as low as 1.5 mg/L
Action?	*Patient toxic and levels raised:*
	• If life-threatening, i.e. level >4 mg/L, omit drug, treat with Digibind
	• Determine cause before restarting
	• If restarting, consider a lower dose. In general, to achieve a serum concentration of half the value, reduce the maintenance dose by half
	Patient toxic but levels within therapeutic range:
	• Exclude other causes of toxic symptoms
	• Check K$^+$
	• Reduce dose, consider additional therapy for cardiac failure of arrhythmia
	Patient clinically undertreated, and levels low:
	• Increase dose, usually by 50–75 mcg, and recheck levels
	Patient clinically undertreated, but levels within therapeutic range:
	• Consider additional therapy
Important	Hypokalaemia and hypothyroidism are commonly associated with digoxin toxicity, so in suspected toxicity, check K$^+$ and thyroid function!

Drugs That Can *Increase* Digoxin Levels

• Macrolides	• Itraconazole
• Quinidine	• Telmisartan
• Amiodarone	• Diltiazem
• Propafenone	• Ciclosporin
• Bendroflumethiazide	• Furosemide
• Verapamil	• Spironolactone

Drugs That Can *Reduce* Digoxin Levels

• Antacids
• St John's Wort
• Colestyramine

Phenytoin

Table 37.3 TDM for Phenytoin

Loading dose	Loading dose 20 mg/kg (max. per dose 2 g) Maximum rate of 50 mg/min
Maintenance dose	100 mg every 6–8 hours (by intravenous infusion or by slow intravenous injection or by mouth) adjusted according to plasma-concentration monitoring. Doses can be split if not tolerated
Why?	Ensure achieving therapeutic target Avoid toxicity (primarily neurological symptoms, e.g. confusion, nystagmus, ataxia, depressed conscious states and seizures) Narrow therapeutic index A fit-free patient, with no signs of toxicity, requires no levels
When?	Take levels 2–4 weeks after starting the drug or changing the dose For IV regimen: 4–6 hours postdose For PO regimen: trough level predose In an emergency, take levels at any time
Meaning?	Recommended therapeutic range 5–20 mg/L The drug is largely albumin bound, so you might need to adjust for a low albumin: $$\text{adjusted phenytoin level} = \text{reported level}/(0.02 \times \text{serum albumin}) + 0.1$$ If your patient has low albumin, ensure to read the 'corrected phenytoin' level which will consider the free phenytoin. *Note* – feeds can interact with phenytoin, reducing their serum levels. Therefore stop patient feeds 2 hours before and 2 hours after each dose

Action?	*Patient showing toxic signs and level raised or level within range:*
	• Seek expert advice on dose reduction
	
	Patient fitting and levels low:
	• Consider a loading dose:
	
	$$\text{Loading dose (mg)} = 0.67 \times \text{weight in kg} \times \text{change in plasma concentration required (mg/L)}$$
	
	• Increase maintenance dose as follows:
	  • <7 mg/L, increase daily dose by 100 mg OD
	  • 7–12 mg/L, increase daily dose by 50 mg OD
	  • 12–16 mg/L, increase daily dose by 25 mg OD
	
	Patient fitting and levels are in the therapeutic range:
	• Seek expert advice: patient might well need additional/alternative therapy
	• Before you make a dose change, seek expert advice!

Drugs That Can *Increase* Phenytoin Levels

- Amiodarone
- Clarithromycin
- Metronidazole
- Isoniazid
- Fluoxetine

- Trimethoprim
- Chloramphenicol
- Cimetidine
- Voriconazole
- Fluconazole
- Fluvoxamine

Drugs That Can *Reduce* Phenytoin Levels

- Alcohol
- Rifampicin
- Carbamazepine
- Theophylline
- Antacids
- St John's Wort

Theophylline/aminophylline

Table 37.4 TDM for theophylline/aminophylline

Loading dose	5 mg/kg IV over 30 minutes (if not previously treated with theophylline)
Maintenance dose	500–700 mcg/kg/h IV, adjusted according to plasma theophylline levels Oral therapy depends on the brand In the obese patient, use *ideal body weight* to calculate the dose, as aminophylline distributes poorly in adipose tissue
Why?	Ensure achieving therapeutic target Avoid toxicity (vomiting, arrhythmias, seizures) For IV therapy: TDM is essential, as the drug has a narrow therapeutic range For PO therapy: TDM is not generally required unless the patient is clinically undertreated or showing signs of toxicity
When?	IV infusion: take levels at 6 and 18 hours, repeating daily Oral therapy: take trough levels 8 hours post dose (if slow-release preparation), after 2 to 3 days of treatment
Meaning?	Recommended therapeutic range 55–110 mmol/L or 10–20 mg/L

Action?	In most patients, theophylline has linear kinetics, so doubling the dose will double the serum concentration. Look out for the odd patient who breaks the rule.
	Acute patient, with low/high level:
	• Adjust dose by desired fraction
	Acute patient in range:
	• Repeat levels daily
	Chronic patient, with low/high level:
	• Having excluded a reversible cause, adjust the dose
	Chronic patient in range:
	• Suspected toxicity: consider a second drug or pathology causing toxic signs. You might need to stop theophylline regardless
	Symptomatic patient:
	• Consider alternative therapy
Important	Children metabolise theophylline quicker than adults so are likely to require higher doses
	Beware those in whom the theophylline half-life is increased, i.e. those in whom a normal dose may cause toxicity: cardiac failure, liver failure, the elderly, those taking enzyme inhibitors (e.g. cimetidine, ciprofloxacin)
	Beware of those in whom the theophylline half-life is decreased, i.e. those in whom a normal dose may be ineffective: smokers, chronic alcoholics, those taking enzyme inducers (e.g. rifampicin, phenytoin). The effect of smoking can be maintained up to 6 months after cessation

Serum levels predict the type of adverse effects well, but are less good at predicting severity (Table 37.5):

Table 37.5 Adverse reactions with theophylline/aminophylline

Level (mg/L)	Adverse reaction	Frequency
<5	Usually absent	N/A
5–20	Nausea and vomiting	5–10%
20–35	As above + diarrhoea, irritability, arrhythmias	25%
>35	As above + seizures	80%

Vancomycin

Table 37.6 TDM for vancomycin

| Loading dose | • Actual body weight (ABW) is used for loading. Loading dose is independent of a patient's renal function |
| | • Weigh patient (kg) and use table below to select loading dose, volume and duration of infusion: |

ABW (kg)	Loading dose
<60 kg	1 g
60–90 kg	1.5 g
>90 kg	2 g

Maintenance dose
- CrCl is used for maintenance dosing
- Give first maintenance dose 12, 24 or 48 hours after start of loading dose according to the dose interval in the table below:

CrCl (mL/min)	Maintenance Dose	Dose interval	Time of first vancomycin trough level
>110	1.5 g	12-hourly	Before fourth dose
90–110	1.25 g	12-hourly	Before fourth dose
75–89	1 g	12-hourly	Before fourth dose
55–74	750 mg	12-hourly	Before fourth dose
40–54	500 mg	12-hourly	Before fourth dose
30–39	750 mg	24-hourly	Before third dose
20–29	500 mg	24-hourly	Before third dose
<20	500 mg	48-hourly	Before second dose

Why?	Renally toxic and ototoxic at raised levels
When?	Take trough level just prior to next dose, as per table above. Repeat levels either:
	• Daily if renal function is poor
	• Twice weekly if renal function is stable
Meaning?	Predose (trough) 10–15 mg/L
	15–20 mg/L used for less sensitive strains of MRSA and severe or deep-seated infections, e.g. MRSA pneumonia, osteomyelitis, endocarditis, bacteraemia

Action?	Predose (trough) level	Maintenance dose adjustment
	<5 mg/L	Move up to 2 levels from current dosing schedule
	5–10 mg/L	Move up 1 level from current dosing schedule
	10–15 mg/L	Continue at current dose
	15–20 mg/L	Continue at current dose
	20–25 mg/L	Move down 1 level without omitting any doses
	>25 mg/L	Omit next dose and decrease by two levels from current dosing schedule
	>30 mg/L	Seek advice from microbiology

Amikacin

Table 37.7 TDM for Amikacin

Standard dosing	7.5 mg/kg IV BD (max. dose = 750 mg BD; max. cumulative dose = 15 g) Use actual body weight (kg) unless the patient is obese If obese use corrected body weight (CBW)

	Creatinine clearance	Dosing frequency
	>50	12-hourly
	20–50	24-hourly
	<20	Discuss with microbiology or pharmacy

When?	Pre (trough) = immediately before next dose Post (peak) = 1 hour after dose change Check levels after every dose change and repeat twice-weekly unless renal impairment, when they should be checked daily or as advised
Meaning?	*Levels* Pre <10 mg/L Post 20–30 mg/L
Action?	If the *predose (trough)* concentration is high, the interval between doses must be increased. If the *postdose (peak)* concentration is high, the dose must be decreased

Other Drugs

Table 37.8 shows a summary of some other drugs that you might be asked to check levels for.

Table 37.8 TDM for other drugs

Drug	Half-life (hours)	Target range	When to sample	Sampling notes
Carbamazepine	Chronic therapy 5–27	Multiple anticonvulsants 4–8 mg/L Single drug 8–12 mg/L	Predose (trough level) after 2 to 4 weeks on initiation Chronic therapy after 4 days	Aim for higher end of range if monotherapy Half-life decreases with chronic therapy
Lithium	18–36	0.4–1.0 mmol/L	12 hours postdose, 4 to 7 days after starting treatment	Desired level varies with indication
Phenobarbital	120	15–40 mg/L	Predose (trough) after 3 to 4 weeks, due to long half-life	Poor correlation between level and response
Sodium valproate	8–15	50–100 mg/L	Predose (trough level) after 2 to 4 days	Correlation between level and efficacy less reliable

Chapter

38

Drug Hypersensitivities and Contraindications

Roman Landowski

Primum non nocere ('first, do no harm') is a fine principle. However, *any* medicine worth using has a risk of side effects, so it is important to assess the risk/benefit ratio. The manufacturers' data sheets tend to be overly liberal with their contraindications, being written by lawyers. So how do you make your assessment? Use your Pharmacy Medicines Information Centre to understand local and national guidelines and BNF guidance; then you won't have to blindly follow the rules but will be able to use them to guide your particular clinical options.

Enshrined rules and received wisdom tend to fit into one of three categories:

The Good	Sensible advice that you should try to follow
The Bad	Overly cautious advice that you can (usually) flout with impunity
The Ugly	Tricky advice that may appear overly cautious, but you should still follow as there is usually a safer alternative agent

The Good

'Don't give him any NSAIDs – he's got renal impairment.'

Patients with renal impairment rely on renal prostaglandins to maintain their *renal* blood flow – and these are blocked by NSAIDs. NSAIDs will worsen renal perfusion in these patients and precipitate a sudden deterioration in renal function. Liver cirrhosis and heart failure patients might be similarly dependent on prostaglandins to maintain renal perfusion. COX-2 inhibitors (e.g. celecoxib, valdecoxib) are just as bad and you should avoid them all. Use paracetamol, tramadol or opiates as alternative analgesics.

'Don't use NSAIDs in liver failure.'

Bleeding is a common problem in decompensated liver disease and NSAIDs can exacerbate this (antiplatelet effects) or cause bleeding (GI ulcers). In this regard, the COX-2 NSAIDs are better, but they can still cause GI bleeding. Avoid the lot and stick to paracetamol/tramadol for pain and prednisolone for inflammation.

'Avoid morphine and CNS depressants in liver failure.'

The worry here is tipping your patient into hepatic encephalopathy. Remember, though, that the CNS depressant effects of opiates (and of any drug) are dose-dependent. So morphine can be used to treat severe pain in cirrhotics as long as you start at low doses (e.g. 5 mg PO) and increase in small increments, and only as long as they are conscious enough to appreciate it! Obviously with antihistamines try the non-sedating loratadine or cetirizine first, but if you need to use a stronger antipruritic such as chlorphenamine or hydroxyzine then start at half dose and increase as tolerated.

The Bad

'Beta-blockers kill asthmatics.'

Well yes, it can happen, but the risk depends on the degree of $\beta2$-blockade (bronchial effect) that you inflict. Cardioselective beta-blockers (e.g. atenolol, bisoprolol) mainly block $\beta1$-(cardiac) receptors (although you might see asthma exacerbation at high doses). Non-selective beta-blockers (e.g. propranolol, carvedilol) are more likely to cause bronchoconstriction, especially at high doses. You can use beta-blockers safely in non-brittle asthmatics if you stick to the cardioselective ones – start at low doses and watch out for signs of asthma exacerbation whenever you increase the dose.

'Don't use cephalosporins in patients allergic to penicillin!'

OK, cephalosporins and penicillin are both beta-lactams and there is a recognised cross allergy, which the books will tell you is 10%. Half of the problem is that people describe non-immunological reactions such as headache, confusion and diarrhoea as evidence of allergy. They might well be hypersensitivity reactions, but they are not allergic. If the patient is sure that he/she has had a real immunological reaction such as oedema or rash then try to use a non-cephalosporin alternative (e.g. gentamicin for UTIs or clarithromycin for chest infections). Otherwise, check that the emergency tray is in date and crack on with the cefuroxime!

'Aspirin with warfarin is dangerous.'

Correction: warfarin is dangerous however you prescribe it – it features in half of all hospital adverse drug reaction incident reports. Aspirin is sometimes co-prescribed with warfarin for the treatment of arterial atherosclerosis in patients with venous thrombosis. The problem arises when patients self-medicate with

PRN aspirin, as the high doses used for pain relief (e.g. 600 mg QDS) are much more likely to cause bleeds than low antiplatelet doses (e.g. 75 mg OD). Regular antiplatelet aspirin is not without risk, but it is at least predictable, monitorable and reducible (with concomitant omeprazole).

The Ugly

'Better stop the metformin as he is now in renal failure.'

Tricky – does renal failure really increase your risk of lactic acidosis with metformin? A 2003 Cochrane review concluded that the evidence was thin. The trouble is that this very rare side effect has a high mortality (approximately 20–30% depending on degree and duration), and the benefit of the drug probably does not justify the worry involved in prescribing it. Change to a gliptin or pioglitazone or just ask the patient to inject insulin.

'Young girls can't take metoclopramide.'

There is an element of truth in this. Teenage girls seem to be particularly prone to extrapyramidal reactions caused by dopamine antagonists such as metoclopramide. These Parkinsonian reactions are not dangerous, but they are distressing for the patient. Of course, most girls *will not* have this reaction and, as it is dose-related, you can try using a half dose first. Still, the whole point of giving metoclopramide is to stop nausea, which is less likely to occur if you are using homeopathic doses, so it is easier to just use cyclizine or ondansetron.

'Don't give aspirin to asthmatics.'

Aspirin is said to set off asthma in about 5% of asthmatics and, although this effect is dose-related, it often occurs at low doses (an average of 69 mg in one study). If the patient has had previous aspirin or NSAIDs without bronchoconstriction, then you can be sure they won't react now. If you are starting low-dose aspirin in a patient who is unsure whether he/she has had aspirin or NSAIDs before, start at a quarter of a 75 mg tablet for the first dose, then half a tablet and then a full tablet on day 3. If there are any problems, use clopidogrel.

Likewise, if you need immediate antiplatelet effects then give a loading dose (300 mg) of clopidogrel and then titrate up the aspirin. NSAIDs show the same problem as aspirin, but COX-2 inhibitors are safe, so you may use celecoxib if your asthmatic patient needs an anti-inflammatory.

The Ridiculous!

'He can't have penicillamine as he's allergic to penicillin.'

Yes, penicillamine is a breakdown product of penicillin and yes, the spellings are quite similar, but no, penicillamine does not have a beta-lactam ring and cross-hypersensitivity is very much the exception rather than the rule.

Interactions that Matter

Roman Landowski

39

The man lay on our renal ward, too weak to rise, limbs aching, new bedsores burning and his transplant failing. Two lines on his drug chart explained why: (i) ciclosporin 100 mg BD (but he had been on that uneventfully for years); (ii) recently started simvastatin 20 mg ON. And there it was – iatrogenic rhabdomyolysis from a simple drug interaction.

How do Drugs Interact?

Pharmacokinetic Interactions

- *Enzyme inhibition* – e.g. as above, ciclosporin inhibits the simvastatin-metabolising cytochrome P450 3A4, causing simvastatin levels to double and the risk of (level-dependent) rhabdomyolysis to rise.

- *Enzyme induction* – e.g. rifampicin can induce P450 C9, which metabolises warfarin. Result? Halving of warfarin levels and reducing the INR to ineffective levels unless the warfarin dose is doubled. Unlike enzyme inhibition, which occurs soon after the interacting drug is added, the effects of enzyme induction can take a couple of weeks to become maximal.

- *Reduced absorption* – e.g. calcium taken with ciprofloxacin binds to form an insoluble chelate, lowering ciprofloxacin blood levels. Avoid by leaving a 2-hour time gap between the drugs.

- *Competition for renal excretion*, raising levels of each drug – e.g. probenecid raises amoxicillin levels when treating endocarditis (500 mg QDS amoxicillin + 500 mg QDS probenecid).

- *Drug displacement from protein-binding sites* (usually on albumin) is rarely of clinical consequence. Valproate can displace phenytoin from albumin-binding sites, but the rise in free phenytoin is temporary as it is free phenytoin that is cleared. Since a greater amount is available for clearance, the free phenytoin will return to normal (although it will be a larger proportion of the total phenytoin that itself will have fallen).

Pharmacodynamic Interactions

In these interactions, two drugs either have opposing effects on the same receptor (e.g. propranolol and salbutamol on bronchial β2 receptors) or they share common side effects (e.g. ciclosporin and simvastatin independently cause an increased risk of myopathy – this is a second reason for the interaction in the opening paragraph).

An Approach to Interactions

Appendix 1 in the BNF gives a good list of potential drug interactions. However, they are not all clinically relevant: some are theoretical or are rarely seen in practice (e.g. amiodarone–amitriptyline, digoxin–phenytoin). The serious interactions usually involve those drugs whose levels only need to be increased slightly above their therapeutic range for toxicity to occur. These drugs are commonly monitored (see Chapter 37 – Therapeutic Drug Monitoring). Is your drug one of these? Examples that require monitoring are:

• Amikacin	• Ciclosporin
• Digoxin	• Lithium
• Phenytoin	• Gentamicin
• Theophylline	• Warfarin

Next, you should check whether any drug that is recognised to cause interactions is prescribed. Examples of these are given in Table 39.1:

Table 39.1 Drugs likely to cause interactions

Enzyme inhibitors likely to increase levels	Enzyme inducers likely to reduce levels
• Erythromycin	• Rifampicin
• Fluconazole	• Phenobarbital
• Diltiazem	• Carbamazepine
• Ciprofloxacin	• St John's Wort
• Ritonavir	

It's back to **SICKLy** – if the drug you intend to prescribe falls into any of these categories then you should actively CHECK for interactions in the following places:

BNF, Appendix 1

Stockley's Drug Interactions

Your ward pharmacist or Pharmacy Medicines Information Centre

In summary, remember your Medicines Information Centre (MIC): if you are prescribing a drug that requires Monitoring, or is known to cause frequent Interactions, then Check to see that no problems are likely to be caused by your new drug interacting with what is already on the patient's drug chart.

Specific Examples

Warfarin has so many drug interactions that it deserves a chapter to itself, so we gave it one (see Chapter 28 – Warfarin Prescribing). For other drugs, the list below details the more common interactions that are both predictable and serious. The drug affected is named first in **bold** with the interacting drug next in *italics*, followed by a summary of the effects, mechanism and recommendations for use in practice.

Alendronate – *Calcium*

Alendronate and other bisphosphonates such as clodronate and **risedronate** work by chelating calcium in bone, where they inhibit bone turnover. They will also chelate with ingested calcium taken at the same time and so become unavailable for absorption. To avoid this, allow a 2-hour gap between any calcium supplements or milk and the oral bisphosphonate.

Azathioprine – *Allopurinol*

Azathioprine levels increase by a factor of 3–4 after allopurinol is started. This can lead to azathioprine-induced neutropenia and thrombocytopenia (dose related). Allopurinol inhibits xanthine oxidase, which is the enzyme responsible for clearing **azathioprine**. If azathioprine is being started in a patient already on allopurinol, just prescribe one-quarter to one-third of the dose that you would normally have used. Xanthine oxidase also clears **mercaptopurine**, so a similar dose reduction is required when allopurinol is added.

Carbamazepine – *Erythromycin*

Carbamazepine: macrolides (**erythromycin**, **azithromycin** or **clarithromycin**) inhibit carbamazepine metabolism, the levels of which thus rise two- to fourfold. Symptoms of toxicity (ataxia, nausea, confusion and double vision, and AV block) develop over 1 to 3 days. If alternative antibiotics cannot be used, then you should monitor carbamazepine levels and adjust the dose accordingly. Once erythromycin is stopped, the carbamazepine levels will fall over about a week.

Ciclosporin – *Phenytoin*

Ciclosporin levels halve over 2 weeks after phenytoin has been added, necessitating an approximate doubling of ciclosporin dosage. When starting phenytoin in a patient already on ciclosporin, check the ciclosporin levels twice a week and increase dosage gradually as necessary. Continue for at least 2 weeks or until dose requirements even out. The same can occur after **phenobarbital** or **carbamazepine** is started.

Ciprofloxacin – *Calcium*

Ciprofloxacin (and other quinolones, such as **ofloxacin** and **norfloxacin**) levels drop by 30–50% when calcium is taken at the same time, because calcium chelates ciprofloxacin in the gut. So separate administration by at least 2 (and preferably 4) hours. Tetracyclines such as **doxycycline** or **oxytetracycline** interact likewise and the same rules of separation apply. **Iron** and **antacids** containing **magnesium** or **aluminium** will also chelate tetracyclines or quinolones if taken at the same time, so should likewise be separated. **Milk** can also chelate these antibiotics if given in volumes of greater than 300 mL. The quantities in tea or coffee are unlikely to cause clinical problems.

Digoxin – *Amiodarone*

Digoxin levels are doubled in some patients when amiodarone is added, due to reduced renal clearance. The effects are nausea, bradycardia, arrhythmias and visual disturbances. These can occur over 7–28 days. Take a level at the beginning of treatment and again after 2 and 4 weeks and adjust digoxin doses as necessary. In practice, you would normally halve the digoxin dose immediately upon commencement of amiodarone. If this is done, then it is important to check the digoxin level after a month to ensure that the reduction was warranted.

Digoxin – *Furosemide*

Digoxin toxicity is more likely when patients are hypokalaemic, so beware toxicity (in the face of normal levels) when using potassium-losing diuretics such as furosemide and *bendroflumethiazide*. This problem is less likely if the patient if also taking an ACE inhibitor, an angiotensin receptor blocker or spironolactone as these all raise potassium. Otherwise, it is better to prescribe co-amilofruse (amiloride with furosemide) than furosemide.

Digoxin – *Verapamil* (See Chapter 37 – Therapeutic Drug Monitoring)

Digoxin levels can be increased in a dose-dependent manner by concurrent verapamil. This can cause digoxin toxicity unless digoxin doses are reduced by 33–50%. Verapamil 160 mg OD leads to a 40% increase in digoxin levels, while verapamil 240 mg OD increases levels by 70%. The effect is due to reduced clearance and takes place over 2–14 days. Since verapamil and digoxin share similar slowing effects on the SA and AV nodes, there are increased risks of bradycardia and AV block, even if digoxin levels remain unchanged. Diltiazem is less likely to increase digoxin levels and so would be safer than verapamil.

Lithium – *Diclofenac*

Lithium levels can be raised by 15–60% when *NSAIDs* such as *diclofenac, ibuprofen* or *indomethacin* are added. This is dangerous as lithium toxicity (effects: restlessness, nausea and neurotoxicity) occurs just above therapeutic levels (therapeutic = 0.4–1.2 mmol/L, toxic = 1.5 mmol/L). Toxicity, which develops over 1 to 7 days, is possibly due to NSAID-induced sodium retention, as lithium tends to follow sodium in the kidney. Lithium should be monitored at the beginning and after 1 week of concomitant NSAIDs, or sooner if toxicity is suspected.

Methadone – *Rifampicin*

Enzyme induction means that methadone levels can be halved by concurrent use of rifampicin. To prevent opioid withdrawal, methadone doses should be built up over 2 to 5 weeks to about two to three times the initial dose. Better control can be achieved by splitting the daily dose into two parts to allow for more rapid clearance.

Phenytoin – *Nasogastric feeds*

Oral phenytoin is chelated by nasogastric feeds (but not normal food), resulting in a large but inconsistent reduction in phenytoin absorption, and a fall in phenytoin level. Stopping the feed for 1 hour before and for 2 hours after phenytoin might help. If not, change to IV phenytoin by giving the preferred daily dose of phenytoin split into two to four evenly spread doses (e.g. 300 mg NG OD to 100 mg IV TDS).

Prednisolone – *Rifampicin, Carbamazepine*

Levels of prednisolone and other glucocorticoids such as **hydrocortisone** and **dexamethasone** can be reduced two- to threefold by concurrent rifampicin over 2–14 days (due to enzyme induction). This necessitates a two- to threefold increase in steroid dose over about 2 weeks, and a similar tailing off over 2 weeks once the rifampicin is stopped. Carbamazepine affects steroids in the same way.

Simvastatin – *Ciclosporin*

Simvastatin levels can be doubled by concomitant use of ciclosporin; this can cause simvastatin-mediated myopathy or rhabdomyolysis. Simvastatin can be used as long as the dose is restricted to 10 mg/day. Other statins interact similarly, although less so for **pravastatin.**

Simvastatin – *Erythromycin*

Simvastatin levels can be increased three- to sixfold by macrolides such as *clarithromycin, azithromycin* or erythromycin. These inhibit 3A4 enzymes, which metabolise simvastatin. Symptoms of myopathy appear in 4–20 days, and it is most simple to stop the statin for the duration of the antibiotic course.

Simvastatin – *Fluconazole*

Simvastatin and **atorvastatin** levels can be increased by the triazole antifungals *fluconazole* and *itraconazole* (enzyme inhibition), leading to a risk of myopathy. For short courses of antifungals, stop simvastatin or atorvastatin for the duration. For long courses (over a month), switch to pravastatin.

Tacrolimus – *Erythromycin*

Erythromycin (and *clarithromycin* and *azithromycin*) raise tacrolimus levels by four- to sixfold over 3 days, resulting in tacrolimus toxicity (including renal damage). Levels return to normal just as quickly after erythromycin is stopped, but unless you want to be taking daily tacrolimus levels it is better to swap to another antibiotic (e.g. doxycycline). **Ciclosporin** is similarly affected when given with these macrolides.

Theophylline – *Ciprofloxacin*

Theophylline levels can be rapidly increased two- to threefold by concurrent ciprofloxacin due to enzyme inhibition. Symptoms of theophylline toxicity (see erythromycin) may well ensue unless theophylline or **aminophylline** doses are halved at onset of ciprofloxacin. Norfloxacin has less of an effect while ofloxacin and levofloxacin do not interact.

Theophylline – *Erythromycin*

Erythromycin and other macrolides such as *clarithromycin* and *azithromycin* will inhibit the 3A4 enzymes that metabolise theophylline, leading to a 25–40% increase in theophylline levels after 3 to 5 days. Once the antibiotics are stopped, it takes about 2 days for theophylline to fall back to its previous level. Check levels at the beginning of therapy, and if they are near the top of the range (>80 mmol/L or 15 mg/L) then shave 25% off the dose of theophylline for the duration of the antibiotic course. Otherwise, continue with the normal dose unless symptoms of toxicity (e.g. tachycardia, agitation and nausea) occur, in which case withhold theophylline and take levels. The same goes for **aminophylline**.

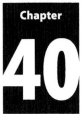

Infections

Peter Wilson

Choice of antibiotic should be dictated by spectrum of activity, tissue penetration, potency and cost, and local patterns of infection in your hospital. Too much to remember? Check your smartphone formulary app or ask your microbiologist, who will have written a local antibiotic policy (e.g. 'What is first line for hospital-acquired pneumonia?'). If a patient is ill enough to have required admission for the treatment of an infection, the *route of administration* should generally be IV. This ensures that adequate plasma levels are achieved independent of gastrointestinal absorption. The *dose* should always be checked in the BNF.

TOP TIPS

- Take microbiological specimens *before* starting treatment.
- Base your initial choice of antibiotic on the most likely pathogen(s).
- In the critically ill, use the highest IV dose, but not the IM route.
- Be familiar with the *Control of Infection Manual* and the *Hospital Formulary* (usually smartphone app).
- Microbiology and infection control staff are usually available on 24-hour call. Use them!

If in doubt, seek advice. The microbiologists welcome clinical queries – this can prevent a lot of problems later on.

Acute Meningitis

RED ALERT

DO NOT DELAY TREATMENT, particularly if outside a hospital – do not wait for a lumbar puncture or CT scan. DO try to get blood culture first.

- Covering *S. pneumoniae, H. influenzae, N. meningitidis*: ceftriaxone 2 g IV 24-hourly
- For patients with a history of anaphylaxis to penicillins and/or cephalosporins: chloramphenicol 1 g PO/IV 6–8-hourly
- For contacts: prophylaxis required:
  - *N. meningitidis*: ciprofloxacin PO one dose or rifampicin PO BD for 2 days
  - *H. influenzae*: ciprofloxacin PO BD for 3 days or rifampicin PO BD for 4 days

---

TOP TIPS

If there is no venous access, give ceftriaxone IM (in more than one site) for the *first dose only*.
- Contact the on-call microbiologist for treatment advice.
- DO NOT administer antibiotics intrathecally.
- Treatment should be modified according to microbiology results.

REMEMBER, this is a notifiable disease: you MUST contact microbiology, who will arrange prophylaxis for all household and institutional contacts.

Antibiotic Treatment
Upper Respiratory Tract Infections
These are generally viral and do not usually require antibiotics.

   Remember, amoxicillin + glandular fever = rash and unscathed virus.

Acute Streptococcal Pharyngitis
- If admitted: benzylpenicillin IV 6-hourly
- If an oral regimen is to be used: benzylpenicillin IM for 1 dose, then amoxicillin PO 8-hourly for 10 days
- If penicillin-allergic: erythromycin PO for 10 days

Acute Otitis Media
- *S. pneumoniae, H. influenzae*
- First choice: amoxicillin PO 8-hourly for 5 days

   Or

- Co-amoxiclav PO 8-hourly for 5 days
- If penicillin-allergic: erythromycin PO for 5 days.

Lower Respiratory Tract Infections

- Lobar pneumonia in a younger person should be treated more aggressively if there is deterioration on oral agents.
- Empyema is serious. It requires immediate large-bore drainage ± surgery. Get specialist advice at once.
- Give antibiotics as soon as pneumonia is diagnosed.
- Use IV treatment if the patient has two of:
  - Respiratory rate ≥30/min
  - Diastolic BP ≤60 mmHg
  - Blood urea ≥7 mmol/L
- Clarithromycin causes less GI hurry than erythromycin.

Community-Acquired Pneumonia

- Usually susceptible to first-line antibiotics (Table 40.1).
- If not severely ill, cover *H. influenzae*, *S. pneumoniae* and atypicals: amoxicillin IV 8-hourly plus clarithromycin IV 12-hourly.
- If severely ill, use highest recommended dose IV: first choice – cefuroxime IV 8-hourly plus clarithromycin IV 12-hourly.
- Duration of therapy: 7 days (may be longer if Legionella, staphylococcal or Gram-negative bacilli pneumonia are suspected or confirmed; discuss with microbiology).
- Post-influenza: cover for *S. aureus* as above. Cover against *S. aureus* should be adequate with clarithromycin but change to high-dose flucloxacillin if confirmed.
- *Mycoplasma* or *Chlamydia* spp. suspected: clarithromycin or doxycycline.
- Legionnaire's suspected: consult microbiologist urgently!

Infective Exacerbation of COPD

- Usually viral, but difficult to distinguish from bacterial.
- Change in sputum colour or volume, or if pyrexial: amoxicillin PO 8-hourly (consider IV for first 48 h).
- If penicillin-allergic: doxycycline PO 12- to 24-hourly.
- More severe exacerbation/poor response to agents above: doxycycline or co-amoxiclav PO.

Aspiration Pneumonia

- Only use antibiotics if signs of infection.
- Often mouth flora, i.e. anaerobes and microaerophilic streptococci: co-amoxiclav IV or PO 8-hourly.
- If penicillin-allergic: clindamycin 300 mg PO 6-hourly.

Hospital-Acquired Pneumonia

- Onset >72 hours after admission.
- Often coliforms, which can be multiresistant: first choice – cefuroxime IV 8-hourly or co-amoxiclav IV or PO 8-hourly.
- If sensitivity pattern warrants (e.g. Pseudomonas *spp.*), or ventilated on ICU: ceftazidime IV 8-hourly or piperacillin/tazobactam IV 8-hourly or ciprofloxacin (use 400mg, not 200mg) IV 12-hourly.

TOP TIPS

- The need for IV therapy should be reviewed after 48 hours.
- If no response to treatment, take advice from a microbiologist and/or chest physician.
- Remember to consider TB, HIV infection and underlying diseases such as lung cancer.

Gastroenteritis

- Antibiotics should usually be avoided and can prolong excretion of the pathogen. They should be used in typhoid, septicaemic infections or AIDS.
- For other infections, antibiotics should be reserved for the severely ill, immunocompromised or elderly.
- The most important aspect of treatment is oral rehydration with glucose electrolyte solutions (or salty soups and fruit juices) and complex carbohydrates (promote active glucose/sodium co-transport).
- Avoid opiates and loperamide.
- Typhoid: first choice – azithromycin PO 24-hourly or ceftriaxone IV 24-hourly.
- Salmonella, Shigella: first choice – ciprofloxacin IV or PO 12-hourly; alternatives – azithromycin PO single dose.
- Campylobacter (treatment often ineffective): first choice – azithromycin PO 24-hourly; alternative – ciprofloxacin PO 12-hourly.
- Amoebiasis –avoid steroids:
  - Metronidazole or tinidazole (single dose at night).
  - Diloxanide furoate – on expert advice only.
- Giardia: metronidazole or tinidazole.
- Yersinia: seek expert advice.
- Cryptosporidiosis: seek expert advice.

Clostridium difficile (Pseudomembranous Colitis)

- The most common infective diarrhoea in hospital.
- Induced by many different antibiotics, the most common being clindamycin, although most antibiotics can be implicated.
- Stop all antibiotics if possible.
- If treatment of a concurrent infection is essential, use an antibiotic least likely to worsen diarrhoea, e.g. ciprofloxacin or vancomycin.
- Persisting or severe symptoms: first choice – vancomycin 125 mg PO 6-hourly (can predispose to emergence of vancomycin-resistant enterococci); alternative – metronidazole PO 8-hourly (stop before 2 weeks of therapy, as risk of peripheral neuropathy).

TOP TIPS for Managing *Clostridium difficile*

- If patient is unable to take medication PO, give metronidazole IV 8-hourly (Note: IV vancomycin is not effective).
- Persistence of toxin is not a guide to treatment duration.
- Usually, treat established pseudomembranous colitis until diarrhoea stops.
- Surgery might be required. Relapses are common.

Soft-Tissue Infection (Cellulitis)

- Administer IV antibiotics without delay for any spreading cellulitis.
- Oral treatment is reserved for localised or minor infection.
- First choice: benzylpenicillin IV 6-hourly + flucloxacillin IV 6-hourly. Switch to oral when clinically appropriate.
- No IV access: clindamycin PO 6-hourly.
- Penicillin allergy: clindamycin PO 6-hourly.

RED ALERT

- Blistering, dusky purple or black discoloration suggests necrosis requiring surgical intervention.
- Necrotising fasciitis is a surgical emergency: seek immediate surgical review – DO NOT wait until the morning!

Urinary Tract Infection

- Upper UTI: give IV antibiotics for 48 hours, then PO for one week.
- Lower UTI: oral treatment for 3 days only. Recurrent infections require longer courses of treatment for 2 to 6 weeks.

- Complicated infection (e.g. anatomical abnormality of renal tract): treatment courses should be for 5 to 7 days.
- Do not treat asymptomatic, elderly or catheterised patients.
- Sexually transmitted diseases can cause similar symptoms, so collect a urinary specimen before treatment whenever practicable.

Uncomplicated, Community Acquired
- Treat only if symptomatic.
- First choice: nitrofurantoin PO 6-hourly.
- Alternative: trimethoprim 200 mg PO 6-hourly.

Hospital Acquired
- First choice: nitrofurantoin 50 mg PO 6-hourly.
- Alternative: ciprofloxacin 500 mg PO 12-hourly.

In Pregnancy
- ALWAYS treat, even if asymptomatic.
- Seek advice from an obstetrician ± microbiologist.
- Cefadroxil PO 12-hourly or amoxicillin PO 8-hourly.
- AVOID trimethoprim in the first trimester and nitrofurantoin in the last trimester.

Bacterial Endocarditis
- Always consult the on-call microbiologist. DO NOT try to treat this condition without advice.
- Three separate sets of blood cultures should be taken before starting treatment.

Septicaemia
- Treat immediately. Patients can succumb to Gram-negative bacteraemia if not adequately treated within 12 hours. The urinary, biliary and respiratory tracts are the most likely sources.
- Initially: cefuroxime IV 8-hourly .
- If patient deteriorates further: add gentamicin IV.
- If allergic to cephalosporins: ciprofloxacin IV 12-hourly + gentamicin IV.
- If suspect anaerobic sepsis: add metronidazole IV 8-hourly.

Neutropenic Sepsis

- Untreated, these patients deteriorate fast – a single spike of fever is sufficient. Hit Gram-negative pathogens first, then after 24 hours staphylococci and, after a further 24 hours, fungi.
- CHECK YOUR LOCAL HOSPITAL PROTOCOL.
- The protocol will usually include broad-spectrum antibiotics with activity against pseudomonas, e.g. piperacillin/tazobactam, ceftazidime, ciprofloxacin.
- If fever is associated with flushing of the Hickman line or redness/discharge around the line exit site, add vancomycin or teicoplanin. Think about taking the line out.

MRSA

MRSA can be four times more invasive than methicillin-sensitive *S. aureus* and difficult to treat because it is usually resistant to several families of antibiotics. Deep surgical wound infections are particularly troublesome. Prolonged treatment with glycopeptides combined with rifampicin, fusidic acid or gentamicin, depending on susceptibility, is effective in some cases, but surgical debridement is often needed. Metal or plastic work must be removed for cure.

Multidrug-Resistant Gram-Negative Bacteria

Infections due to carbapenem-resistant organisms are increasing in hospitals and are difficult to treat. Consult the microbiologist.

Antibiotic Prophylaxis

General Principles

- In most surgical specialties, antibiotic prophylaxis has been shown to be effective in reducing postoperative wound infections (Table 40.1).
- It is not needed in minor clean procedures, e.g. simple hernia repair, removal of lipoma or insertion of central venous or peripheral vascular catheters.
- Parenteral antibiotics should be given with induction of anaesthesia before skin incision. Tissue levels will then be sufficient to kill the bacteria.
- Antibiotics given more than 4 hours after surgery are NOT effective prevention.
- A single large dose of antibiotic is sufficient, except in vascular, and head and neck surgery.
- Use a different antibiotic to treat infection from the one used for prophylaxis.

TOP TIPS

- Ensure administration is always documented (medicolegal).
- Adjust dose if patient is obese.
- Do not give with premedication as timing is variable.
- Check if the patient has had any recent infections with resistant organisms.
- Eradicate MRSA carriage using topical therapy (chlorhexidine, mupirocin nasal ointment) before surgery or, if emergency, during perioperative period.

Table 40.1 Antibiotic prophylaxis

Gastrointestinal procedures	
Appendicectomy	Cefuroxime and metronidazole IV
	If appendix acutely inflamed or pus found, continue with cefuroxime IV 8-hourly + metronidazole IV 8-hourly for 5 days
Colorectal surgery	Cefuroxime + metronidazole IV
Biliary tract surgery:	
Normal bile duct, no stents	No prophylaxis needed
Cholecystectomy, biliary tree involvement, common duct stones	First choice: cefuroxime
	Alternative: co-amoxiclav
	Penicillin allergic: ciprofloxacin
Previous biliary surgery	Add gentamicin IV to the above
Anaerobes suspected e.g. carcinoma	Add metronidazole IV to cefuroxime
	No need to add metronidazole to co-amoxiclav
Upper GI surgery	Cefuroxime IV plus metronidazole IV
Vascular procedures	
	First choice: cefuroxime IV
	Penicillin allergic: clarithromycin IV
	Second choice: co-amoxiclav 1.2 g IV at induction
	MRSA: teicoplanin or vancomycin
Gynaecology	
Hysterectomy, emergency C-section	First choice: cefuroxime IV
	Penicillin allergic: clindamycin IV plus ciprofloxacin IV
Termination of pregnancy	Uncomplicated: no prophylactic antibiotic
	History of PID: doxycycline 100 mg BD for 14 days postoperatively

Orthopaedic procedures

Compound fractures	Cefuroxime IV at induction, then IV 8-hourly for three doses
Joint replacement and spinal surgery	First choice: cefuroxime IV at induction, then (if prosthesis inserted) IV 8-hourly for two doses
	Penicillin allergic: clarithromycin IV at induction, then (if prosthesis inserted), clarithromycin PO at 12 hours
	For revision of infected joint replacement, start specific treatment rather than antibiotic prophylaxis
	For repeat operations due to infection, gentamicin cement should be incorporated at operation
	Metronidazole is NOT indicated for routine orthopaedic prophylaxis

Urology procedures

Mid-stream urine culture must be checked before and during surgery

Transurethral resection of prostate	First choice: gentamicin IV
	Second choice: ciprofloxacin 500 mg PO 1–2 hours before procedure

Deprescribing

Katherine Le Bosquet

What is Deprescribing?

The English Deprescribing Network define deprescribing as:

> *A collaborative process, with the patient and/or their carer, to ensure the safe and effective withdrawal of medicines that are no longer appropriate, beneficial or wanted, guided by a person-centred approach and shared decision-making.*

Patients want to be on the right medications to treat their problems and, following discussion, are usually happy to stop taking those that are no longer working or needed, or if they are causing more harm than benefit. Deprescribing is the job of everyone who prescribes.

It is important to avoid stopping medications without:

- speaking to the patient
- generating an action plan
- documenting the change and the rationale in the notes.

(If acting on instruction and you don't know why … ask! The pharmacist will inevitably ask why a medication was stopped and won't accept the answer 'my consultant said so.') This will save your colleagues hours of time when writing discharge letters. GPs and primary care teams need this detail to continue the patient's care in the community, and to understand if a medication can be restarted if required or if there was an adverse event or treatment failure.

Failure to adhere to these simple guidelines causes a loss of the patient's trust, and confusion once discharged back to the community.

Questions to Ask When Prescribing New Medications or Stopping Medicines

1. Has anyone spoken to the patient or carer about changing their medication?
2. Do you have the full medication list available? Has medicines reconciliation been completed and actioned?

3. Have you stopped the medications identified as not working when starting new medication?

4. Have you looked through the full medication list before starting a medication, to make sure that it is not on there already?
   (You would be amazed how often this happens!)

5. If initiating a second-line treatment, have you checked that they were adherent to the first-line treatment, and if they were, has the dose been increased to the maximum available dose?

6. If the medication is for a short duration or you want it to be reviewed after a certain time, have you documented this? i.e. two-week trial of .... then ....

7. Does this medication need to be weaned or can it just be stopped?
   (Your ward pharmacist can help you with this.)

Think about what you say to the patient! If we stop telling patients a medication is 'for life' on initiation, then it will be easier to change when the patients' circumstances or co-morbidities change. Clinicians who have tried to stop a medication and struggle with the complexities of withdrawal tend to dislike prescribing that medication again in the future.

Discharge Letters Following Medication Review

Questions to ask and things to do:

1. Have you included details of the medication changes made during the admission? If the GP is to start .... and to stop .... never assume that someone else knows when to stop a medication.

2. If medications have been stopped, include any follow-up or monitoring required in the discharge letter.

3. Be realistic with GP follow-up. Have you given enough information? e.g. GP to review furosemide .... for what reason? Swollen ankles, wet cough, low BP, AKI, patient adherence etc. What is the target you were aiming for? Do you want it to be weaned off or increased to max. tolerated dose?

4. Be realistic with the timeframe. Will the GP take bloods in 2 days and review if you put it in the letter? Will it even be seen in 2 days? Have you told the patient or in urgent cases rung the GP and arranged this follow-up?

5. Did the patient tell you something about their medication that the GP or community team need to know i.e. 'My house is full of medicines and I get confused', 'I can't open those eye drops my pharmacy send'.

Errors in discharge letters are ten a penny for GP practices. If changes are not clearly documented, the prescriber will often revert to the original dose assuming it was an error, undoing all your good work. Conversely patients where only the 'key medications for this admission' were listed may have all their regular medications stopped as the GP labours under the false impression that 'the hospital must have reviewed and stopped them'.

Be aware of the importance of the discharge letter as they are the only communication that the primary care team receives about the time spent in hospital by your patient. Try rereading your letters before sending, or swap with a friend; ask yourself – could you continue care with this information?

Electronic Prescribing

Samrina Bhatti

Reviewers: Ann Slee, Barry Jubraj and
Caroline Anderson

This chapter will focus on ePrescribing in hospitals: although there are some similarities with primary care, significant differences exist. While electronic prescribing has many safety advantages, it also introduces new issues and risks. Here are some to be aware of:

Logging In and Out

Your system administrator should provide you with ePrescribing login details. Don't share these with anyone and log out after each use: you will be held accountable for others using your details.

Allergies and Intolerances

Before prescribing a medication, consider and record potential allergies and intolerances to it on the ePrescribing system (even if this means entering 'status is not known') and the nature of the reaction. Sometimes, these are entered by other multidisciplinary team (MDT) members – so look before you prescribe.

Clinical Decision Support

Different ePrescribing systems provide varied levels of clinical decision support (CDS), perhaps prompting you with alerts, e.g. to complete a venous thromboembolism assessment, to check allergies, consider potential drug–drug interactions or prevent duplicate prescribing. CDS can also help with weight- or height-based dose calculations. However, understand the scope and limitations of CDS before using it, and avoid over-reliance on CDS as it may fail to warn you about potential errors. In some cases, it may be appropriate to override the CDS. If you choose to do this, clearly document your decision in the patient record.

Medication Dictionaries

Most ePrescribing systems have in-built medication dictionaries and formularies. These may be locally configured and will vary depending on the system you are using.

Different nomenclature for medicines should be considered before prescribing. For example, if 'vitamin K' doesn't appear in the drug dictionary, try a different name for the same substance i.e. 'phytomenadione'. *If you are unsure of the nomenclature for the medication you require, liaise with the clinical team managing your ePrescribing system.*

Most systems will also have a 'blank order' form available which will allow you to prescribe medications which are not currently listed in the drug catalogue. This should only be used when absolutely necessary because this action may bypass any CDS provided by the system.

Brand-Only Prescribing

Generic medications have the same active pharmaceutical ingredient as one another but may have different brand names. For example, paracetamol is the generic name for the branded medications Calpol® and Panadol®. Certain generic medications must be prescribed by brand only, for reasons including:

- Differing bioavailability for different preparations e.g. Tacrolimus preparations (Adoport® and Advagraf®)
- Lack of interchangeability of some modified-release (MR) e.g. Nifedipine MR preparations (Adalat LA® and Nifedipress MR®)
- Varying inhaler potency e.g. Beclometasone dipropionate inhalers (Clenil Modulite® and Qvar®).

Therefore, these should be searched for or chosen by brand name when being prescribed electronically.

Preconfigured Selection

Some ePrescribing systems allow you to select from a preconfigured list of commonly prescribed medications with their typical associated dose, strength and frequency. The frequency may include 'when required', 'once only', regular or a predefined course. There may also be options to bulk prescribe two or more medications from prebuilt protocols for certain conditions (usually based on locally or nationally agreed prescribing protocols). This may help reduce prescribing errors by reducing the number of medications which need to be prescribed individually.

Common Errors

When prescribing long-hand, you may search a medication with the first three letters of the prescription and select the incorrect medication, e.g. select metronidazole instead of metformin, or an inadvertent finger slip of adding that extra '0' leading to an incorrect dose of '400 mg' instead of '40 mg'. Picking from drop-down menus and auto-populated prescriptions can also result in incorrect selections of look-alike-sound-alike drugs.

Indications

Include the correct indications for certain groups of medications so that they can be appropriately reviewed by other members of the MDT. Entering this information accurately can also help organisations monitor prescribing and compiling 'secondary use of prescribing' reports. The ePrescribing system may have a mandatory or optional field to record this information.

Transferring From Previously Entered Data

There may be an option to automatically transfer across medications from a previous inpatient episode or from a medicines reconciliation that has been verified by a pharmacist. This can save time and minimise transcribing errors, but a thorough medication review should be undertaken before using 'automatic transfer' because some medicines may need to be stopped, held or adjusted.

Pathology Data

The ePrescribing system may not automatically link to the pathology system. You must therefore review pathology results before prescribing, as this may affect your decision to prescribe a particular medication or dose.

When prescribing medications that require therapeutic drug monitoring (see Chapter 37 – Therapeutic Drug Monitoring), you may need to enter the time and date of the associated pathology test into the system (for example, blood drug levels for vancomycin). This will help to ensure further doses are prescribed appropriately. Many ePrescribing systems have direct links to local policies and guidelines that can help guide you further.

Transferring Between ePrescribing Systems

There may be more than one system used for ePrescribing in a single hospital, for example, one for inpatients on general wards and a different system for the intensive care unit. If the systems are not interfaced (directly linked), careful transcription between systems will be necessary as patients move between clinical areas. Particular attention is required to 'suspend' and 'unsuspend' medications on the ePrescribing systems. Reconciliation across systems is recommended on transfer.

Likewise, you may be transferring a patient to a ward that does not have an ePrescribing system, in which case similar transcription safety principles apply to paper drug charts. When amending a medication, make sure you check for any associated prescription notes (for example, administration instructions or review date). There might be important information which should be carried forward onto the new prescription.

When creating new electronic prescription orders, you should consider and understand the most appropriate place to record relevant information for other members of the MDT. This may be within the electronic prescription itself or in an entirely different place.

Omitting Doses

Where a medication needs to be omitted for a short period of time (e.g. pre- or postsurgery) you may be able to 'suspend' electronic medication orders or 'omit' particular doses. This is most appropriate where there is a clear timeframe in which doses are to be omitted and a clear rationale to restart. For example, when co-prescribing a 5-day course of clarithromycin alongside the patient's regular simvastatin, you may decide to withhold five simvastatin doses due to an interaction. The system may allow you to 'omit' the particular doses or 'suspend' the prescription without needing to 'cancel' or 'discontinue' the simvastatin. This avoids the risk of inadvertent omission of simvastatin on day 6 because the prescription would be automatically reactivated.

Finally, it is important to note that some hospitals are still using paper medication charts and others may have a mixed economy of both paper and electronic prescribing (particularly as hospitals transition wholly to the use of ePrescribing systems). Therefore, some prescribing might still occur on paper supplementary charts (common examples include blood products, insulins and warfarin). It is important to ensure that you account for any paper charts and incorporate ALL medications into your prescribing-related decisions. Do not assume that everything is visible in one place or on one system.

Chapter 43

Corticosteroids
Robert Shulman

Converting from one steroid to another is often necessary and can cause much head scratching. But help is at hand with Table 43.1.

As an example, hydrocortisone 50 mg IV QDS can be converted to prednisolone 50 mg PO OM.

Table 43.1 Steroid conversion

Drug	Equivalent anti-inflammatory dose (mg)
Betamethasone	0.75
Cortisone acetate	25
Deflazacort	6
Dexamethasone	0.75
Fludrocortisone	Mineralocorticoid, so no anti-inflammatory activity
Hydrocortisone	20
Methylprednisolone	4
Prednisolone	5
Prednisone	5
Triamcinolone	4

Management of Steroid Therapy

To maximise the benefit and minimise the risk of corticosteroids therapy, think of the following:

- Use the lowest possible dose for the shortest length of time.
- Steroid tablets given in the morning and on alternate days can reduce adrenal suppression.
- Night-time doses can cause insomnia, so try not to prescribe a dose later than 6 pm.

Withdrawal of Corticosteroids

Some situations require gradual withdrawal of systemic corticosteroids to avoid relapse of disease and adrenal failure. These include when the patient has:

- recently taken repeated steroid courses (particularly if taken for longer than 3 weeks)
- taken a short course within 1 year of stopping long-term therapy
- other possible causes of adrenal suppression
- received >40 mg daily prednisolone (or equivalent)
- taken repeated doses in the evening
- received more than 3 weeks corticosteroid treatment.

You can reduce corticosteroid dose rapidly down to the equivalent of prednisolone 7.5 mg daily, but then take it more slowly.

Example

Remembering to be CLEAR with timing, reduce from prednisolone 40 mg OD as follows:

- 30 mg OM for 3 days, then
- 20 mg OM for 3 days, then
- 10 mg OM for 3 days, then
- 7.5 mg OM for 5 days, then
- 5 mg OM for 5 days, then
- 2.5 mg OM for 5 days, then stop!

Assess the disease during withdrawal to ensure that relapse does not occur and watch for symptoms of adrenal failure, which might include:

- Fatigue
- Weight loss
- Skin hyperpigmentation
- Hypotension causing syncopal episodes
- Abdominal pain
- Nausea, diarrhoea or vomiting.

You can stop systemic corticosteroids abruptly in those whose disease is unlikely to relapse, those who have received treatment for 3 weeks or less, and those not included in the patient groups above.

Intravenous Therapy

Robert Shulman

Some Simple Rules!

1. Check that the patient really needs the drug IV and can't have it in some other (cheaper and less risky) way.

2. Don't administer an IV drug until you know how. Check your hospital's IV guide or Medusa (national IV guide: www.injguide.nhs.uk), or try the appendix of the BNF (https://bnf.nice.org.uk)

3. Get a thorough check from someone else before administration. It's been known for doctors, when tired, to read an ampoule as saying 'ampicillin' when it actually says, 'strong potassium chloride'. Never trust yourself. Check the drug, concentration, quantity, expiry data and that you are giving the right drug, at the right dose, in the right diluent, over the right time period, by the right route.

4. Consider whether the IV route should be peripheral or central. See the tips below to take the trauma out of the parenteral route!

Possible Indications for Central Venous Administration

- Hypertonic, concentrated (e.g. KCl IV) or irritant fluids (e.g. cytotoxics, total parenteral nutrition, inotropes)

- Rapid administration of large volumes (e.g. in shock)

- Long-term venous access (e.g. cytotoxics, total parenteral nutrition)

- Administration of drugs with a pharmacological action on veins, such as vasoconstriction (e.g. dopamine, noradrenaline)

- Need to give incompatible drugs at the same time (central lines can have multiple lumens).

Drugs that MUST be administered centrally include adrenaline, noradrenaline (unless your hospital has a local policy), dopamine and amiodarone.

Speed of Administration

Guidelines are there for a reason! Too fast, and …

- furosemide: ototoxicity (deafness) at >4 mg/minute
- fusidic acid: haemolysis and hepatotoxicity
- vancomycin: red man syndrome (flushing, macular rash, fever, rigors), especially if given over <1 hour
- sulfonamides: crystals in the urine
- ranitidine: arrhythmias, arrest
- theophylline: arrhythmias, nausea, vomiting, tachycardia
- potassium chloride: arrhythmias, arrest (generally avoid >20 mmol/h)
- lidocaine: arrhythmias, arrest
- phenytoin: arrhythmias, respiratory/cardiac arrest if administered at >50 mg/minute
- methylprednisolone sodium succinate: cardiovascular collapse at >50 mg/minute.

Problems!

Pain on Injection

Pain can be caused by factors including pH, tonicity and chemical irritancy.

- Check that the drug is the right one. Potassium chloride hurts like hell before it kills!
- Ensure that the drug is going into the vein and not an artery/tissue!
- See if it is a common problem – pain is seen more with erythromycin, 8.4% bicarbonate, glucose at concentrations >10%, phenytoin and vancomycin.

If pain is still a problem, try reducing the rate or increasing the dilution.

Phlebitis

This is a red, inflamed vein, corded (hard), with a low flow of drug solution through the vein. Do not plough on; resite the cannula.

Extravasation (Infiltration, Tissuing)

This is the accidental infiltration of IV fluids/drugs into the subcutaneous tissue. It can cause local inflammation or pain. Mostly, there isn't a problem. However, tissue damage is more likely if the drug is hypertonic (high osmolarity), chemically irritant or has a pH outside 4–8 (i.e. strongly acidic/alkaline). The main culprits in this regard are:

- aciclovir, erythromycin, vancomycin, gentamicin
- calcium chloride, bicarbonate 8.4%, mannitol

- noradrenaline, adrenaline, potassium high concentration, TPN
- phenobarbital, phenytoin, aminophylline
- cytotoxic drugs, radiographic contrast media.

If extravasation occurs, stop the infusion immediately. Avoid flushing the line or applying pressure to the site. Elevate.

Initially, do not remove the catheter/needle – this will be useful to aspirate fluid from the site and to administer an antidote, if needed. If an antidote is not needed, remove the catheter/needle, after aspiration. Subsequent management may include heat or cold packs, antidotes, surgery and local hyaluronidase injection.

Index